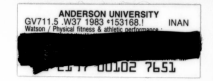

PHYSICAL FITNESS
& ATHLETIC PERFORMANCE

A. W. S. WATSON, 1941-

PHYSICAL FITNESS
& ATHLETIC
PERFORMANCE

A GUIDE FOR STUDENTS, ATHLETES & COACHES

 LONGMAN   London and New York

Longman Group Limited
Longman House
Burnt Mill, Harlow, Essex CM20 2JE, England
and Associated Companies throughout the World.

Published in the United States of America
by Longman Inc., New York

First published 1983

British Library Cataloguing in Publication Data
Watson, A. W. S.
  Physical fitness and athletic performance.
  1. Physical fitness   2. Athletics
  I. Title
  613.7′1   GV436

  ISBN 0-582-49094-4

Library of Congress Cataloging in Publication Data
Watson, A. W. S., 1941–
  Physical fitness and athletic performance.

  Bibliography: p.
  Includes index.
  1. Physical education and training.
2. Physical fitness – Testing.   I. Title.
GV711.5.W37   613.7′1   82-7155
ISBN 0-582-49094-4 (pbk.)   AACR2

Set in 10/12 Linotron 202 Plantin
Printed in Singapore by
Selector Printing Co Pte Ltd

CONTENTS

v

3   FEATURES OF TRAINING, WARM-UP, MOTOR UNIT TYPES

4   TRAINING METHODS

5 EVALUATION OF FITNESS LEVELS

PREFACE

This book is concerned with athletic performance: its biological basis, the factors which influence it, and how it can be evaluated, and then improved, through training. It is the product of a number of years of lecturing on such topics and of advising athletes from a wide variety of sports. This experience has suggested the need for a volume which gives an account of some of the recent research into physical performance, fitness and the effects of training, in a form that is useful to the serious athlete and those who advise him. A number of reviews of the research literature are available but these are often extremely specialised and usually very limited in scope. At the opposite end of the spectrum there is no shortage of 'recipe books' of training exercises. Useful as these are to the beginner, they are inadequate for the serious practitioner and are seldom up-to-date. This volume is an attempt to bridge the gap between these two types of publication and to provide some of the information required by the serious coach and those who work with sportsmen in a professional capacity as teachers, organisers, medical advisers, etc.

The information available on the effects of exercise has increased dramatically over the last few years. In particular, much more is now known concerning the specific effects of different types of training and of the important biochemical changes that occur as a result of physical activity. Some of this recent work challenges many of the traditional approaches to exercise and training, and as more detailed research is carried out it is becoming clear that the effects of conditioning programmes are often more subtle and less general than had previously been supposed. This suggests that the modern exercise practitioner must be prepared to develop his own techniques based on the specific needs of the individual athlete and the activity he is undertaking. If the coach or adviser is to do this effectively, he requires a sound understanding of basic biological principles and the ability to establish the training requirements of the individual sportsman.

It is my pleasure to thank the many people who have contributed to the production of this book. Professor G. R. Kelman, Professor

Risteard Mulcahy, Dr Dan McCarthy and Dr Richard O'Flaherty have read parts of the manuscript and have provided valuable assistance in particular areas. My thanks are also due to other individuals too numerous to mention by name: friends, students, colleagues, coaches and athletes who have given me the benefit of their specialist knowledge of particular sports and training methods – and I hope I have learned something from them; however, the errors which remain are my responsibility, and the views expressed are my own. Finally, I am most grateful to all those who assisted so skilfully in the production of the illustrations, and to Eileen Healy for her secretarial assistance.

TONY WATSON
Wimbotsham, Norfolk

1 COMPONENTS OF PHYSICAL PERFORMANCE

INTRODUCTION

It is paradoxical that in the age of the micro-chip, when many routine tasks are being taken out of human hands, there would seem to be an increasing interest in physical performance and training. This is expressed in a number of ways: more people may be engaging in physically active leisure pursuits as a reaction to the increasing mechanisation of society. In the realm of international sport there is much more emphasis on preparation and training, and many of the so-called amateur sports are now effectively full-time occupations. All this activity receives a good deal of attention by the media and, indeed, many popular fitness programmes are actually initiated and organised by various sections of the press. Certain aspects of training physiology have almost become part of general culture and terms that would have been obscure to many physiologists a few years ago are now used, not always correctly, on radio and television and in the popular press.

Opportunities for the systematic study of sport have also increased and courses are now available in such areas as sports science, recreation, sports medicine, exercise physiology and biochemistry, and sports psychology. A good deal of research is now being carried out in many of these fields. The aims of this type of work include investigation of the differences between average and outstanding athletes and the improvement of training methods.

The most outstanding characteristic of the champion athlete is that he wins. In many other respects he may well be quite ordinary or even somewhat substandard. Sports science examines performance in relation to the individual achieving it, and then attempts to discover the reasons for the success. It then seeks to translate these findings into a form that will be useful to others – often by suggesting improvements in training methods. Superficial observation of the athlete may, or may not, provide some clues about his performance. The individual is quite likely to be aged between 20 and 35. He could well have a striking

1

physique – lean and streamlined or perhaps large and heavily muscled. Perhaps his behaviour is unusual – exceptionally outgoing and agressive; or he may appear introverted and withdrawn. Do these characteristics make a contribution to performance or are they purely incidental and irrelevant? If the individual is a champion shot-putter, is this due to an exceptional level of skill or to great strength? If it can be established that the athlete is exceptionally strong the investigator will want to know the aspects of anatomy and physiology this can be attributed to and whether they are innate characteristics or have been acquired through training.

Techniques from several different disciplines have been used to answer such questions. These include: physiology, anatomy, biochemistry, genetics, physical anthropology, mechanics, psychology and sociology. This book is concerned with contributions arising from areas at the start of the list. In particular, no attempt is made to review the many significant advances made in the area of sports psychology. The importance of this area is acknowledged, but it is outside the scope of this book and the reader is referred elsewhere for information.

FACTORS INFLUENCING PHYSICAL PERFORMANCE

At the most general level physical performance is a function of all the physical and mental characteristics of the individual. Some of these are determined at the moment of conception by the genetic material derived from the father and mother. The most obvious is the individual's gender. Some characteristics may be acquired later through the processes of growth, maturation and learning, while others result from the interaction of the individual's basic genetic make-up with his environment. All this may seem rather far removed from the scoring of goals in a football match or the winning of an athletic event, but in fact such achievements are subject to just these constraints. Sporting achievement is a complex mixture of genetic make-up and environmental influences – including training – and in attempting to reach any meaningful conclusions about physical performance it is useful to try to separate these two factors. There have been several studies of genetic effects in athletes and it is becoming clear that they have a most important influence (see pp. 75–6). In the case of a few characteristics – most obviously gender – the effect is entirely genetic. But in many others there is interaction with environmental factors such as training. Training can 'fine tune' the characteristic, but the limits of achievement are genetically predetermined.

Certain environmental influences occurring after conception have permanent effects and, together with genetic factors, these represent 'invariable' constraints on the athlete's performance. Characteristics that are relevant to physical performance and over which the individual has little or no control include gender, age, somatotype, height, and the distribution of motor unit types. Many of the effects of the first two factors are obvious, but a few of the lesser known points are referred to elsewhere. 'Physique' is briefly considered later in the chapter and 'motor unit distribution' is discussed in Chapter 3.

At a less general level it is possible to demonstrate that physical performance is influenced by specific physiological characteristics, many of which can (at least in theory) be measured or otherwise described. These include such variables as strength, joint mobility (flexibility) and the capacity for various types of physical work (endurance). These are frequently classified as components of *physical fitness*. This, too, is a useful way of analysing physical performance because it highlights variables which can generally be modified or improved through training. As more is known about the biological effects of exercise it has become clear that the changes are all due to definite anatomical, physiological and biochemical adaptions. It seems convenient to group these variable aspects of physical performance under one heading since they are all factors over which the individual has some control. In this book they are considered as components of fitness and their biological basis is discussed in Chapter 2.

Chapters 3 and 4 are concerned with the effects of training. Considerable difficulties are enountered when writing in this area as sportsmen trained long before physiology became fashionable and much of the available information has been acquired by trial and error rather than by the processes of science. When scientific investigations were started they tended to concentrate on matters occurring *during* exercise, and it is only recently that carefully controlled studies have been made of the merits of different training methods. Some of the most useful information available about training has come from such studies but they are few in number and, due to the nature of scientific investigation, are limited in scope. The investigations are usually of short duration because it is very difficult to ensure that individuals train under controlled conditions for long periods. And they have to be confined to one particular kind of subject – quite often, college students. It must be a matter of speculation as to how far the results of such studies can be applied to other types of subject. In particular, it is difficult to be sure they will relate to the élite athlete who is already highly trained and whose invariable physical characteristics are unlikely to be average. Although controlled studies on such an individual are theoretically possible, they are, in practice, extremely difficult to organise.

Another problem is the uneven coverage of different areas. A good deal of work has been carried out on endurance training – some on strength, but very little on many other aspect of fitness.

Because of these difficulties the approach to the sections on training is different from that adopted in Chapter 2. I have taken the view that the athlete is not going to wait to begin his training until all the research has been completed, and have tried to make comments on all the major areas. Where possible these have been based on carefully controlled experimental studies, but where such information is not available I have made use of the best information available.

A training programme is most likely to be beneficial if it is specifically designed to meet the individual sportsman's needs. Thus some kind of evaluation of the fitness levels of the athlete is necessary, and this topic is considered in Chapter 5. As with the work on training methods, the information available is less complete and up-to-date than that which exists on basic physiology. Although a large number of general tests have been described, many were developed before the highly specific effects of training were fully appreciated. There is a need to adapt many of these for use with particular types of athlete. The field is so wide that it is impossible to consider all the tests necessary in different situations. I have therefore described tests with general applications and have tried to include material which may help the reader to develop more specific techniques of his own.

PHYSIQUE

Physique has an important influence on athletic performance but is only to a very limited extent under the individual's control. A large number of studies have shown that successful sportsmen tend to have particular types of physique and that this is related to athletic success (for example, see Tanner 1964 and Khosla 1978).

SIZE

Apart from the obvious observation that height is an advantage to rugby forwards, basketball players and throwers, there are also more subtle effects of differences in body size. These occur because the human is three dimensional. If the height of a three-dimensional object is doubled its surface area increases four times and its mass is multiplied eight-fold. Thus, when individuals of different size are considered, the body surface area and the cross-sectional area of muscle (and therefore strength) tend to vary in proportion to the square of height. Variables such as weight and blood volume increase in line with height cubed. Thus changes in size tend to produce differences in the relationships between such variables as strength, weight, power output, acceleration and work capacity. This means that individuals of various sizes are better equipped for different types of activity. A detailed analysis of the mechanical and physiological consequences of changes in size has been made by Asmussen and Christensen (1967) and some of this work is summarised in Table 1.1.

SOMATOTYPE

Somatotyping – a system of classifying individuals on the basis of body shape – was developed by Sheldon during the 1940s and 1950s (Sheldon 1940, 1954). The method is based on the assumption that every phys-

Table 1.1 The influence of body size on some physiological functions and aspects of human performance. Body shape is assumed to remain constant

Function	Proportional to	Effect on the function of increasing height by a factor of 1.5	Example or comment
Body surface area	Height^2	× 2.25	Body surface area increases at a faster rate than height
Body weight	Height^3	×3.375	Weight increases at a much faster rate than height
Body surface area per kg body weight	1/height	×0.67	Better heat conservation in large individuals – an advantage in activities where cold is a problem. Better heat dissipation in small individuals. Preserves cardiac output – an advantage in endurance activities
Blood and lung volumes	Height^3	×3.375	
Strength	Height^2	×2.25	Strength increases at a faster rate than height
Work-rate	Height^3	×3.375	Larger individuals have a much higher work-rate
Anaerobic power	Height^2	×2.25	
Ability to accelerate external object	Height^2	×2.25	Large size an advantage to throwers
Ability to accelerate own body	1/height	×0.67	Large size is a disadvantage in activities where acceleration is important
Lifting own body weight	1/height	×0.67	Size is a disadvantage
Running at constant speed on the level	1	None	Size has no influence
Running up hill	1/height	×0.67	Size is a disadvantage
Long jump	1	None	Size has no influence
High jump	1	See comment	Size has no influence on the trajectory of the jump but extra height raises the centre of gravity which is an advantage

ique can be described in terms of the contribution of three basic components: *endomorphy, mesomorphy* and *ectomorphy.* Features of individuals extreme in each of these three components are listed in Table 1.2.

The Sheldon somatotype is concerned with body shape only. It is not influenced by size. Secondly it is a genotype; that is, it assesses genetically determined aspects of physique that are invariable and not capable of change. Sheldon described somatotype as 'a trajectory or pathway through which the living organism will travel under standard conditions of nutrition and in the absence of grossly disturbing pathology'. It is thus that part of physique which does not change with age, nutrition or the state of training. It is important to appreciate this point. Endomorphy is not the same as being fat and mesomorphy is not simply a measure of muscle bulk. If an endomorph is starved he remains an endomorph even though he may have little or no fat. This is because the basic characteristics of physique which determine his somatotype remain unchanged. Weight training may increase muscle bulk but it does not change the genotype. This point has been demonstrated in a study on the effects of weight training reported by Tanner (1952). It was found that although muscle girths increased, the somatotypes of the subjects remained unchanged.

The individual's actual shape at a given point in time is known as his 'phenotype'. It can be quantified by taking anthropometric measurements such as skinfold thicknesses and muscle girths. In some circles the term 'somatotype' is used to describe the phenotype. This is incorrect usage and leads to considerable confusion. The word 'somatotype' should be reserved for assessments of physique made according to the Sheldon method.

Somatotype has an important influence on physical performance. In a comprehensive study carried out at the 1960 Olympic Games, Tanner

Table 1.2 Characteristics of individuals with extremes of endomorphy, mesomorphy and ectomorphy

	Endomorphy	*Mesomorphy*	*Ectomorphy*
Ratio of weight to height	Initially high and increases with age, becoming very high	High	Low
Head	Spherical; often small in relation to the trunk	A more cubical shape than the head of the endomorph; large in size	Angular, often with a beak-like nose and receding chin
Neck	Short and usually thin in relation to the trunk	Thick and massive	Long and angular
Trunk	Abdomen large in relation to thorax	Thorax large in relation to abdomen	Both abdomen and thorax small in relation to height
	Hips wide in relation to shoulders	Shoulders wide in relation to hips	Both shoulder and hips narrow in relation to height
	Depth large in relation to width	Width large in relation to depth	Both depth and width small in relation to height
Limbs	Arms and thighs large in relation to calves and forearms	All segments massive, the forearms and calves especially so	All segments slender
Wrists and ankles	Small in relation to elbows and knees	All bone sizes large	All bone sizes small
General shape	Spherical	Square, cubical	Linear, angular
Muscle mass	Low	Moderately high in young individuals, then high	Low
Fat content	Increases rapidly with age	Low	Low

(1964) found that less than half the somatotypes present in the general population were represented among Olympic athletes. In addition, it was found that distinctive types of physique were associated with particular events. It has also been shown that a number of physiological variables, such as aerobic capacity and strength, are related to somatotype (Cotes *et al.* 1969; Watson and O'Donovan 1976b, 1977a).

2 COMPONENTS OF PHYSICAL FITNESS

In this chapter the biological basis of the various components of physical fitness is considered. Particular emphasis is placed on aspects relating to the effects of training and some of this material is further developed in Chapters 3 and 4.

FLEXIBILITY

Flexibility is concerned with the movement that occurs at joints. The majority of writers use the term to indicate the range of movement that is possible, and this is the meaning adopted here. Occasionally the term is used in the context of 'freedom of movement', or in other senses. Various uses of the term 'flexibility' are considered at the end of the section.

Most machines require a rigid framework upon which to operate. In the human body this is provided by the skeleton which acts like a series of girders against which the muscles contract and develop force. Many man-made machines are expected to produce only a single kind of movement and so require few movable joints. The human body is capable of an enormous repertoire of different movements and has only a few immovable joints but a large number that are capable of different kinds of motion. Some – e.g. the knee and elbow joints – are designed to move mainly in one plane. These act in a similar manner to the hinge on a door. Others are capable of movement in several directions. Typical examples are the joints found at the hip and shoulder. The structure of a generalised joint is illustrated in Fig. 2.1.

Where two bones come in contact they are covered by a layer of **hyaline cartilage**, a tough, smooth material which reduces friction. The **joint space** is enclosed by the **joint capsule**, a tissue which secretes **synovial fluid**. This is a thick, slippery liquid containing the complex carbohydrate, **hyaluronic acid**, which keeps the joints lubricated. The joint capsule is surrounded by ligaments. These are strong fibrous tissues which prevent the joint being pulled apart; they influence the

Fig. 2.1 Diagram illustrating the general features of a movable joint.

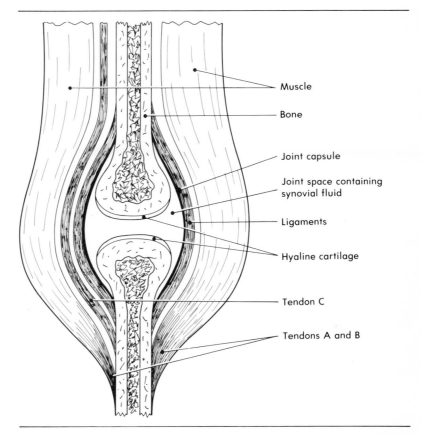

Muscle

Bone

Joint capsule

Joint space containing synovial fluid

Ligaments

Hyaline cartilage

Tendon C

Tendons A and B

range of movement. The knee joint has strong ligaments at the side and back but none at the front. This is reflected in the type of motion possible. The shoulder joint has much looser ligaments which allow a wider range of movement including rotation. Over the ligaments there is a layer of muscle or tendon. Tendons join muscle to bone and may be short, like A and B in Fig. 2.1, or long enough to traverse several joints, such as C, or those that connect the forearm muscles to the finger bones.

Joint motion is limited by a number of factors. Disease and injury can cause changes which include damage to the cartilage, deposits of solids in the joint space, inflammation of the capsule, or a deficiency of synovial fluid. These conditions frequently make any degree of movement painful and difficult. In the healthy individual the range of movement is usually limited by bone structure, the properties of the ligaments, the length of muscles or tendons, or the intervention of soft tissue. Extension of the knee is limited by the length of ligaments at the rear, while flexion is stopped by the contact of soft tissue in the calf and thigh. In contrast, hip flexion is usually limited by the length of the hamstring muscles. The difference is illustrated in Fig. 2.2.

The length and suppleness of ligaments and muscles is not fixed. Where these factors limit joint motion, flexibility can be increased

Fig. 2.2 *Top*: Flexion of the knee is limited by contact between the soft tissue of the calf and thigh. *Bottom*: In contrast, hip flexion is limited by the length of the hamstring group of muscles. This constraint is reduced when the knee is flexed and the hip joint can then be moved much further.

through training. Typical examples are movements at the shoulder, hip, ankle and spine. Two types of change occur. Short-term changes, which follow 'limbering-up' exercises or a warm-up, are quickly reversed. Several weeks of stretching manoeuvres will produce longer lasting changes. These are largely independent of the 'warm-up' phenomenon and a period of limbering-up will produce a further improvement.

STABILITY AND FLEXIBILITY

Joints must be sufficiently flexible to allow the athlete necessary move-

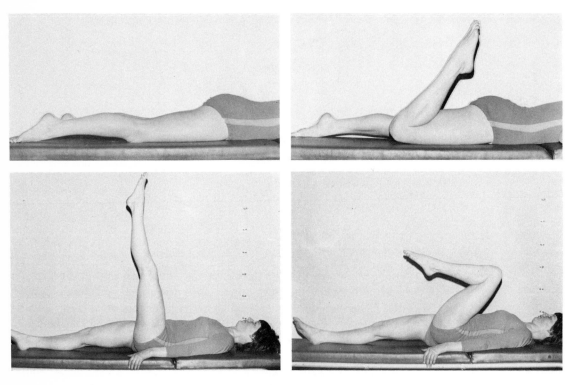

ment, but not so loose that ridigity is lost or a limb put in a position where it is susceptible to injury. Too much flexibility, or flexibility in the wrong place, can be a disadvantage.

Excessive mobility is most commonly a problem at the shoulder and knee. It occurs because the relevant ligaments are too long and results in susceptibility to injury. This is most likely to occur in contact sports such as soccer or rugby. Instability of the shoulder predisposes the individual to dislocation; weak knee ligaments are likely to lead to knee sprain or damage to the semi-lunar cartilage. Both these injuries can be very disabling. A full account of each is given by O'Donoghue (1970). Excessive mobility of the knee or shoulder is a reason for excluding an individual from a heavy contact sport. These conditions can usually be improved by building up the musculature around the joint through weight training. (In cases where the movement is excessive, an orthopaedic surgeon should be consulted.) Studies by Leighton (1957a, 1957b) have shown that many groups of athletes have lower shoulder mobility than some untrained individuals. This is presumably due to a development of the muscles round the shoulder girdle.

Where joint motion is limited primarily by muscle length the situation is different. Too much flexibility is unlikely to lead to instability but too little will result in muscle strain. Hip flexion, illustrated in Fig. 2.2., is a good example. Sprinters are often disabled by hamstring injury which could be prevented by better hip mobility. In order to minimise the possibility of strains, all athletes should aim for a reasonable level of trunk, hip and ankle flexibility. There may then be other requirements specific to particular events.

It is difficult to make generalisations about flexibility because of differences in joint structure and the demands of various sports. Untrained individuals tend to be deficient in most aspects of joint mobility and a general, all-round programme is needed at the commencement of training. Excessive flexibility is unlikely to be a problem at this stage and shoulder exercises are desirable. Although excessive mobility can be a problem in sportsmen, tightness of the shoulder muscles is more common in the untrained and this can lead to muscle strain. Trunk and hip mobility are also important and should be stressed in a general fitness programme. It has been reported that flexibility exercises are sometimes effective treatment for lower back pain, neuromuscular tension and muscular pain (Billing and Loewendahl 1949; Kraus and Raab 1961; De Vries 1974).

Athletes should begin training with a general flexibility programme, paying particular attention to joints where mobility is limited by muscle length. These include the hip, ankle and shoulder and all aspects of spinal motion. There will then be requirements specific to individual sports. A rugby player will need stability at the knee and shoulder; in a javelin thrower shoulder mobility is of greater importance. The coach will need to analyse individual activities to arrive at the combination of rigidity and mobility appropriate to each.

DEFINITIONS

The term flexibility has been used to indicate *the range of motion at a joint*. **Static flexibility** is the range of motion when the joint is moved very slowly. During a rapid movement the range may be slightly different and we would designate this **dynamic flexibility**. Some authors have used the term to describe the resistance of a joint to motion (De Vries 1974) but we prefer the term *resistance* for this variable. The resistance to motion varies with the joint angle, generally being lower near the middle of the range, and with the speed of movement. It has been measured in animals under laboratory conditions (Wright and Johns 1960; Johns and Wright 1962) but not in humans in sporting situations. In a particular motion resistance will be influenced by the action of antagonist muscles, tissue interia and viscosity, as well as the frictional properties of the joints involved. In view of the complex nature of resistance it is not clear whether its measurement would provide information of value to the coach or trainer.

STRENGTH

In the present context strength is the maximum force that can be developed during muscular contraction. Force is measured in the same units as weight – often in lb or kg. Sometimes lb-wt is used instead of lb and kg-wt or kp instead of kg. The latter terms are more correct, but for measurements made on the earth's surface there are no practical differences between the two types of unit.

MUSCLE

There are three types of muscle in the body, each with slightly different properties. **Cardiac muscle** occurs in the heart and is especially suited to short, regular contractions. The gut and blood vessels contain **smooth muscle** which can operate with the minimum of intervention from the nervous system. The third type is that which moves the bones of the skeleton and is known as **skeletal** or **striated muscle**, from its appearance under a microscope. Skeletal muscle is the only type under voluntary control, being operated mainly by the conscious part of the brain. In this book the word *muscle* is used to mean skeletal muscle unless another type is specified.

The gross structure of skeletal muscle can be observed in the lean portion of a joint of meat. It consists of reddish fibres separated by **connective tissue** which is non-contractile. At each end this tissue forms the tendons which join the muscle to bone and transmit the force of contraction.

Connective tissue also isolates the fibre from its neighbours so that each is capable of contracting independently. Muscle also contains several different kinds of nerve, and blood vessels which supply oxygen and nutrients and remove waste products.

The nerves that initiate muscular contraction are known as **motor neurones** (Fig. 2.3). Most control several muscle fibres which contract simultaneously when the nerve is stimulated. The muscles fibres controlled by a single nerve are known as a **motor unit**. Where very precise movement is necessary, such as in the muscles which control the direction of the eyes, each motor unit consists of only a few muscle fibres. In the muscles of the legs and back, motor units may consist of more than 100 fibres. The individual fibres making up a motor unit are widely scattered throughout a particular muscle. Any given portion of a muscle may contain fibres from 20 to 50 different motor units (Burke and Edgerton 1975).

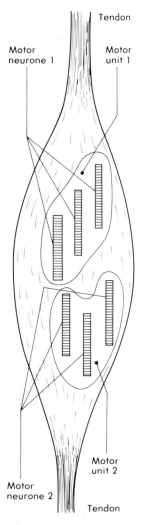

Fig. 2.3 Two motor units distributed inside a muscle.

Tendon

Motor neurone 1

Motor unit 1

Motor unit 2

Motor neurone 2

Tendon

Fig. 2.4 (a) Spatial and (b) temporal summation in muscle. The force developed depends both upon the number of motor units stimulated and the rate of stimulation.

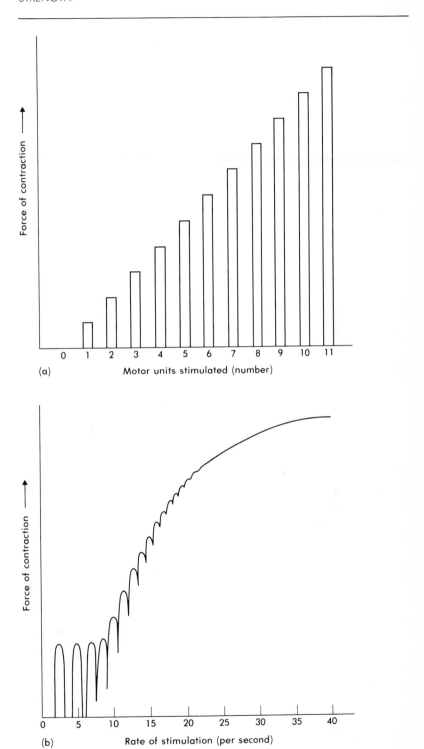

(a) Motor units stimulated (number)

Force of contraction

(b) Rate of stimulation (per second)

Force of contraction

A muscle fibre either contracts maximally or not at all. It is not possible to vary the force of individual contractions of a single fibre but this can be done in a whole muscle in one of two ways: by varying the number of motor units involved in the movement, or by changing the rate at which contraction occurs. These mechanisms are known, respectively, as **spatial** and **temporal summation** and are illustrated in Fig. 2.4.

Although the contraction of skeletal muscle is generally initiated by the conscious part of the brain there is also a degree of automatic control. This often overlooked but it has an important influence upon coordination and the development of strength. The athlete makes the decision to lift a weight or kick a ball with the conscious part of his brain, but the details of motor unit involvement are determined at lower levels of the brain and in the spinal cord. The upper brain acts like a managing director making a policy decision. The detailed execution of this is left to many other individuals who have specialised knowledge of the working of different departments. The overall success of the policy will depend upon the performance of all these individuals. A similar situation occurs with muscular contraction. The nervous system must learn to utilise the available equipment most effectively if maximum strength is to be developed. This process appears to take place in the initial stages of strength training. Several studies have shown that neurological changes take place (e.g. Komi and Buskirk 1972; Komi et al. 1978; Edgerton 1976) and that at the start of training strength increases without a corresponding change in muscle size (Lesmes et al. 1978a). This is presumably due to better utilisation of the existing tissue by the nervous system.

These subconscious mechanisms are influenced by information from several sources, including the muscles themselves. Some of the neural outputs from muscle and other sources are illustrated in Fig. 2.5.

Nerve endings in muscle detect compression, lack of oxygen, excessive tension and other conditions likely to lead to damage. Endings in tendons are sensitive to stretch – an indication of excessive muscle tension. These outputs are fed into the spinal cord and brain, along with information from other sources, and may limit or inhibit muscular contraction. The output from tendons has a direct inhibiting effect upon the motor neurones of the muscles that are causing the tension. This normally prevents the muscle contracting with its maximum force. In exceptional circumstances, such as an extreme emergency, these constraints may be removed. There have been a number of reports of mothers managing to lift huge weights in order to save a trapped child. In laboratory studies exposure to hypnosis, drugs and rifle shots have been shown to produce supra-normal peaks of strength (Ikai and Steinhaus 1961).

In sporting situations acts of strength are seldom the work of single muscles. Usually, several muscles cooperate in the direct development of force, and many others are involved indirectly in stabilising the

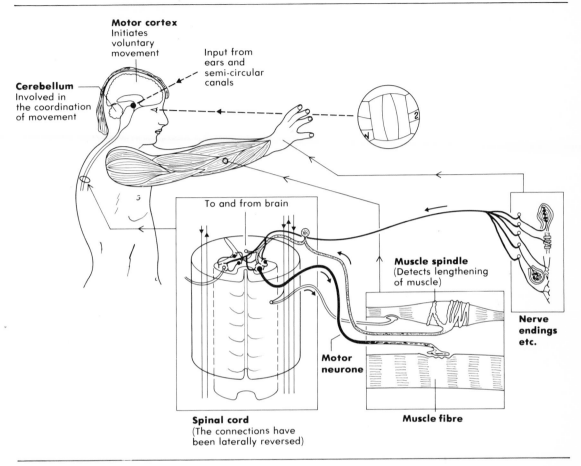

Motor cortex
Initiates
voluntary
movement

Input from
ears and
semi-circular
canals

Cerebellum
Involved in
the coordination
of movement

To and from brain

Muscle spindle
(Detects lengthening
of muscle)

**Nerve
endings
etc.**

**Motor
neurone**

Spinal cord
(The connections have
been laterally reversed)

Muscle fibre

Fig. 2.5 Some of the factors controlling the contraction of skeletal muscle during physical activity. The brain receives sensory information from a variety of sources including the eyes, ears and semi-circular canals, stretch receptors in muscles and tendons, nerve endings in joints and skin. Much of this information is processed in the spinal cord and lower brain and never reaches the level of consciousness.

body. The nervous system has a considerable role in the development of strength and this can be optimised through training and practice.

TYPES OF MUSCULAR CONTRACTION

The term **contraction** is applied to a muscle whenever it is stimulated and consumes energy in developing a force. Rather confusingly, the muscle does not necessarily become shorter in the process. The type of contraction where shortening does occur is known as **concentric** contraction. Sometimes a muscle *contracts* but is unable to overcome a greater opposing force and the muscle gets longer. This type of contraction is termed **eccentric**. It is frequently used to resist the force of gravity as when an individual steps off a chair or lowers a fragile television set onto a table. Occasionally a muscle contracts against the resistance of an immovable object or meets an exactly equal opposing force. In this situation no movement occurs and the contraction is said to be **isometric** because the muscle does not change its length.

Isometric contraction would appear a somewhat pointless phenom-

15

enon but it is actually of great importance as the only means of providing rigidity to the body. The skeleton is a freely movable framework which is stabilised by the contraction of opposing muscles on opposite sides of joints. A heavy weight can be lifted with the arms only if the spine and leg joints are stabilised by isometric contraction. In an isometric contraction no force is wasted in overcoming inertia or tissue resistance, so that a greater force can be developed than in an isotonic contraction.

An **isotonic** contraction occurs if a muscle contracts while maintaining constant tension. It takes place if an isolated muscle is used to lift a weight. Isotonic contractions are rare when a muscle is in position in the body even if a constant weight is raised. This is because the changing length of lever arms varies the resistance applied to the muscle. This is explained in Fig. 2.10. Although the weight of the barbell does not change during the course of a lift, the changing length of lever arms means that the force applied to the muscle does vary. The exercise is not truly isotonic, and the muscle is not developing maximum tension throughout its whole range of movement.

Fig. 2.6 *Left*: most man-made machines operate against a rigid framework provided by immovable joints. *Right*: in man rigidity is provided by the isometric contraction of opposing sets of muscles. In this illustration isometric contraction maintains the stability of the legs and trunk while a weight is being moved with the arms. (courtesy E. J. M. O'Sullivan)

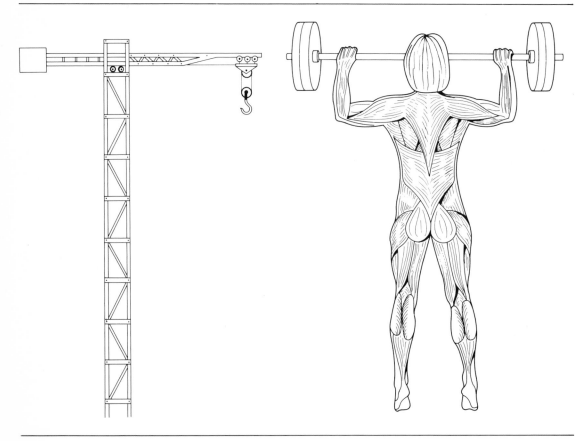

MECHANISM OF MUSCULAR CONTRACTION

Muscle fibres are composed principally of two proteins – **actin** and **myosin** – with smaller amounts of two others – **tropomyosin** and **troponin**. It is the interaction of these four substances that is responsible for the contraction of muscle and the consequent development of force.

When seen under a microscope, skeletal muscle has a characteristically striped appearance. The bands are known as **striations**. This is due to the overlap of two different kinds of protein filament, as illustrated in Fig. 2.7 During the process of contraction the thinner filaments slide over the thicker ones making the muscle shorter and altering the appearance of the striations.

Fig. 2.7 The ultra-structure of muscle: *Above*: the microscopic appearance of a skeletal muscle fibre in the relaxed state. The striations are due to the overlap of the thick and thin filaments. *Below*: the changes that occur when the muscle contracts.

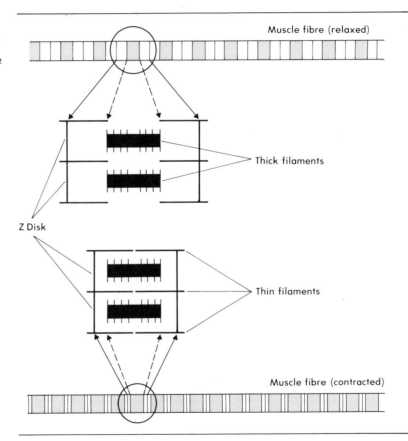

The thick filaments are made up of myosin and contain a series of projections known as **cross-bridges**. The thin filaments are composed principally of actin with small amounts of the other two proteins which play a part in the initiation and control of the contraction process. The necessary energy for contraction is obtained from a high-energy compound, adenosine triphosphate (ATP), which is considered in some detail in the section on endurance. Muscle contracts by the following process. ATP is joined to the myosin cross-bridges which then attach themselves to the actin of the thin filaments. Energy from the ATP enables the cross-bridges to 'flick over' to a different angle, which normally results in movements of the thin filaments. If the muscle is prevented from shortening, an isometric contraction occurs. The process is illustrated in Fig. 2.8.

Fig. 2.8 *Above*: structure of the thick and thin filaments in skeletal muscle. *Below*: Action of the cross-bridges during muscular contraction (see text).

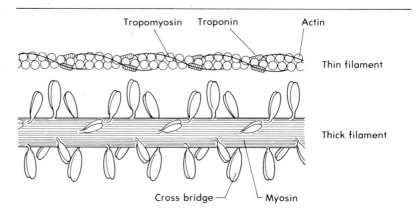

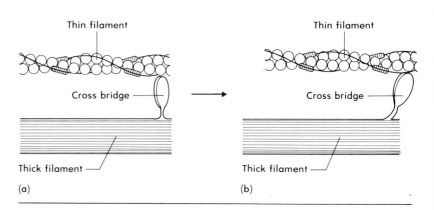

Tension is developed at points where the myosin cross-bridges interact with the actin filaments. It is clear from Fig. 2.7 that the number of such interactions will vary with the position of the two filaments and hence the length of the fibre. As a result, the maximum tension that can be produced by a muscle depends upon its resting length. This is known as the **length–tension relationship** which is illustrated for an isolated muscle in Fig. 2.9. When in place in the body the maximum resting length of most muscles corresponds to that which produces maximum tension. Although the changes in length that occur when a muscle is in position in the body are not as great as those shown in Fig. 2.9, the variations are sufficient to result in significant changes in tension. In the case of most muscles the tension is reduced as the muscle shortens from its resting length.

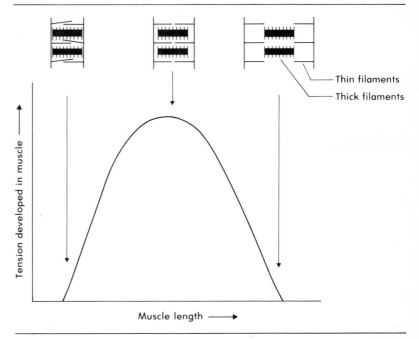

Fig. 2.9 The length–tension relationship of skeletal muscle.

When the muscle is used to move a limb or external object the situation is further complicated by changes in body mechanics. The muscle exerts its maximum force along its axis of contraction. In other directions the resultant force is reduced by a factor equal to the cosine of the angle between the muscle axis and the direction in question. This means that in a limb such as the arm, less of the available force is wasted when the elbow is at a right angle because the muscle is contracting in the same direction as movement is occurring at the hand. This is illustrated in Fig. 2.10. The situation is further complicated if the limb is attempting to exert a force in a constant direction, as is often the case. The resultant force is then also reduced by differences in the direction of limb movement and application of force (see Fig. 2.10).

Figure 2.11 illustrates how the force that can be developed during flexion of the elbow varies with the joint angle. This is simplified treatment of the actual situation. The joint angle at which a particular limb develops maximum tension varies with its construction. Some typical values are given in Table 2.1. The relationship between force and joint angle has a number of applications. In activities requiring great strength it is obviously important to ensure that the force is applied when joints are at their optimum angle. Figure 2.11 indicates that the subject's maximum force of elbow flexion is 80 kg and that this occurs at a joint angle of 120°. At greater and smaller angles the strength is lower. Consider what would be the maximum weight that could be lifted in the manoeuvre shown in Fig. 2.11. The answer is about 20 kg. Although the subject can develop 80 kg of force at one particular angle, 20 kg is

Fig. 2.10 (a) The maximum force of contraction of the muscle is shown as 100 units.
(b) During a maximum contraction of the muscle 100 units of force are available in the direction of contraction. In other directions the force available is less and is zerrc at 90° to the axis of contraction. (c) The muscle in position in the human arm; the force available at the hand is as shown in (b) above. (d) The force available for lifting a weight is further reduced because of the difference in the direction of the lift and the movement of the limb.
In this figure variations in tension due to changes in muscle length have been ignored.

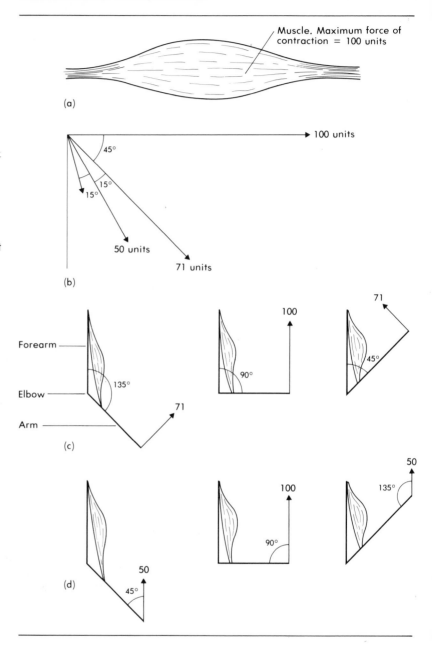

all that can be managed at the end of the range and this will limit the entire lift. This means that maximum strength occurs in an isotonic contraction only at the optimum joint angle.

This phenomenon has implications for strength training where the objective is to stress the muscle by having it work at maximum tension. A maximum isometric contraction will achieve this at one particular joint angle but no movement occurs in this type of exercise and the

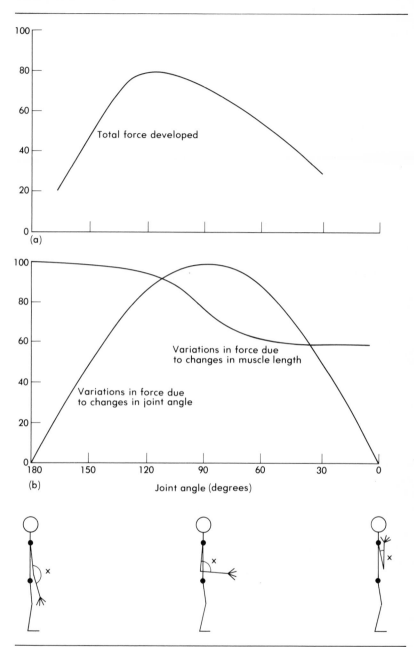

Fig. 2.11 (a) Variations in the total force developed for movement at the elbow. These variations are due to a combination of the two factors illustrated in (b).
(b) The muscle develops its maximum tension when fully stretched (joint angle 180°). At smaller angles the force developed is less, due to the length–tension relationship. The force available at the hand is also reduced by the cosine of the angle between the direction of contraction and the application of the force. These two factors combine to produce the force–joint angle relationship shown in (b).

muscle is trained at only one point in the full range of movement. In order to maintain maximum tension throughout the total range of movement it is necessary to vary the resistance with the joint angle. Machines have been designed which help achieve this by varying the re-sistance to movement by means of a set of weights connected to the limb through a cam. One such weight-training machine is illustrated in

Table 2.1 Angle at which maximum tension is developed in various joints

Action	Joint	Angle at which maximum tension is developed
Forearm flexion	Elbow	120°
Forearm extension	Elbow	Minimum angle
Thigh flexion	Hip	90°
Knee flexion	Hip	160°
Shoulder extension	Shoulder	60°

Fig. 4.5. The extent to which these devices are successful is considered in Chapter 4.

FORCE–VELOCITY RELATIONSHIP

The maximum tension that can be developed in a contraction is influenced by the speed of muscle shortening. Figure 2.12(a) shows the relationship in an isolated muscle that is stimulated electrically. The force is maximum when the speed of contraction is zero, i.e. when the contraction is isometric so that no change in length takes place. If movement *does* occur the force developed decreases as the speed increases. It is thought that this is due to the rate of chemical reactions in muscle being influenced by the mechanical force (Wilkie 1968). Davies (1971) suggests that when a muscle contracts at high speed only a few of the myosin cross-bridges have time to react with actin and, therefore, the tension developed is low.

It is only recently that the force–velocity relationship has been studied in muscle groups operating in position in the human body. The form of the relationship is shown in Fig. 2.12(b). At the higher velocities curves 2.12(a) and 2.12(b) are identical, but in intact muscle the maximum tension is considerably reduced at the lower speeds. This is thought to be due to inhibition in the nervous system that is designed to prevent the overload of tendons (Perrine and Edgerton 1978). The relationship is modified by changes in muscle temperature. A rise in temperature results in an increase in the force developed at a given speed of contraction and in the maximum speed of contraction. Binkhorst *et al.* (1977) report that a 5 degC rise in muscle temperature may result in 10 per cent increase in speed and maximum power output. This is one of the reasons why performance may improve after a warm-up.

The force–velocity relationship of muscle has important implications for sport. Many activities take place at high speed so that performance is influenced by the force that muscles can develop when contracting rapidly. This is not necessarily related to the force that can be produced in a static contraction. It is possible for an individual to have a high level of static strength while being unable to produce much force at high speed. This is illustrated in Fig. 2.12(c). The force–velocity relationship is probably influenced by the individual's motor unit distribution (see Ch. 3) but it can be modified by suitable training (Thorstensson

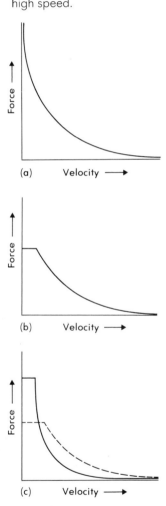

Fig. 2.12 Force–velocity relationship of skeletal muscle. (a) A muscle removed from the body. (b) *In situ* muscle. (c) Curves for one weight-lifter and one jumper. At low speeds of contraction the weight-lifter produces the greatest force but the jumper is stronger at high speed.

(a)   Velocity ⟶

(b)   Velocity ⟶

(c)   Velocity ⟶

——— Weight-lifter
– – – – Jumper

et al. 1977). Lesmes *et al.* (1978a) have demonstrated that when a muscle is trained at constant speed, strength is increased at the training and lower speeds but not at higher speeds. This work means that it is necessary to specify the speed of contraction when describing an individual's strength. For example, in Fig. 2.12(c) the weight-lifter is stronger than the jumper at low speeds but the jumper has the greater strength when the speed of contraction is high. The study of strength at different speeds of contraction has generated a term for contraction taking place at constant speed: **isokinetic contraction**.

ENDURANCE

In everyday language the term 'endurance' is used to describe the durability of an object or an individual's ability to tolerate circumstances that are less than pleasant. In sport it is usually used in the context of the ability to sustain some form of physical activity. This implies that the athlete operates like many mechanical engines which are able to develop maximum power until they finally break down or run out of fuel. In the case of the human machine the situation is less straightforward. The power that can be developed depends upon the duration of the activity. This becomes apparent when the relationship between race length and running speed is examined. There is no particular achievement in being able to run continuously for four minutes; but it is very much harder to do so at a pace which results in a mile being covered. Superficially this may appear to be a matter of speed rather than endurance, but in fact endurance *is* very much involved. A 4-minute mile requires a speed of 6.7 metres per second ($m\ s^{-1}$). It is relatively easy to maintain this pace over 100 metres – the distance would be covered in about 15 seconds, 50 per cent slower than the current world record. A successful miler must maintain this speed for almost 4 minutes which requires the development of half a horsepower over this period. While it is easy to work at this rate for a few seconds, very few individuals can develop such power over a period of several minutes. Endurance thus amounts to more than the ability to continue physical activity; it involves continuing to work at a rate that is high in relation to the duration.

ENERGY SOURCES

Maximum power output varies with duration because different energy sources are involved. Some provide power at a high rate but are quickly exhausted; others last for much longer but are capable of supporting only a low work-rate. There are similarities with a space vehicle that is powered by a multi-stage rocket. The energy available to a well-trained human, from the various sources, are listed in Table 2.2. The size of each energy source is inversely related to the maximum rate of power output. High-energy phosphate compounds provide energy at the

Fig. 2.13 The power output available during activities of various durations. Based on data by Benedict and Cathcart (1913), Wilkie (1959) and other sources.

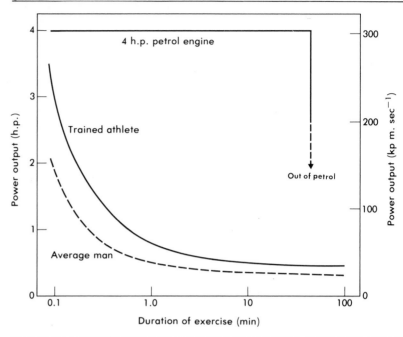

Table 2.2 Energy available to a well-trained athlete from various sources. Values in kcal and *litres of oxygen*

Source	Total energy available	Maximum rate of utilisation (min^{-1})	Time before the source is exhausted at maximum rate of utilisation
Oxidation	30,000	12	40 h
of fats	*6,000*	*2.5*	
Oxidation	3,000	25	2 h
of glycogen	*600*	*5*	
Glycogen →	40	40	1 min
Lactic acid	*8*	*8*	
From	15	90	
high-energy			
phosphate	*3*	*18*	10 s
compounds			

(←AEROBIC→ / ←ANAEROBIC→)

greatest rate but the total amount available is so small that exhaustion occurs in a few seconds. At the other end of the scale the body can have vast stores of fat but the rate of utilisation of this fuel is so low that it is normally used as an energy source only during light or moderate activity. Endurance is primarily about the ability to generate energy at an appropriately high rate. The biological mechanisms by which this occurs are considered below.

Energy for muscular contraction
All the energy used by the human is obtained from foodstuffs, carbohydrates being the most important type. Glucose is one of the simplest

carbohydrates. It is a compound of carbon, hydrogen and oxygen that has a great deal of energy locked into the chemical bonds holding the atoms together. This energy was obtained from the sun during the process of photosynthesis. When glucose is combined with oxygen it is converted back into carbon dioxide and water and the energy in the chemical bonds is released, sometimes as heat, occasionally in a form that can be used to produce muscular contraction. The energy available is known as the **free energy**. In the case of glucose this amounts to approximately 400 kcal per 100 g, about the amount used during one hour of moderately heavy physical activity. If glucose is burnt it is converted into carbon dioxide and water and all the energy is released as heat. It cannot be converted into muscular work and in order to provide energy in a useful form the body allows the reaction to procede in a series of steps. A small amount of energy is released during each step and is transferred to other chemicals that are used during the contraction of muscle. The most important of these is adenosine triphosphate (ATP).

Fig. 2.14 Energy released in a series of steps (a) from water, (b) from glucose, during metabolism in the body.

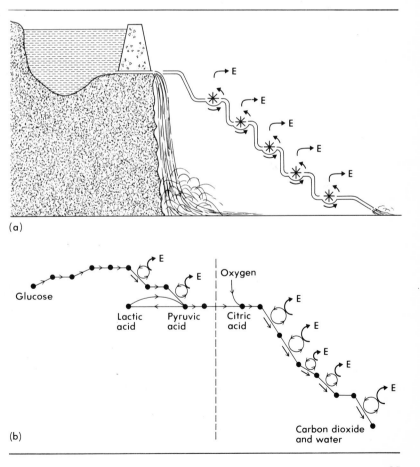

(a)

(b)

The step-wise process occurs due to the intervention of other chemicals known as **enzymes**. These play a vital role in the regulation of all aspects of body chemistry and an introduction to their mode of action will assist in the understanding of several aspects of physical fitness.

ENZYMES

All the energy in foodstuffs and other compounds is locked up in the chemical bonds between atoms. Energy is released when these bonds are broken; it must be taken in before new bonds can be formed. When foodstuffs are converted into carbon dioxide and water the amount of matter remains unchanged but as the bond energy of the products is lower than that of the starting materials, energy is released and becomes available to the body. Unfortunately, it is often difficult to get the process under way. Quite a lot of energy is needed to do this. Before sugar or petrol can be burnt energy must be supplied in the form of a flame or spark. This kind of stimulus is not available in the body and in any case it would serve no useful purpose if the chemical energy in foodstuffs was converted into heat.

The principle role of an enzyme is to assist in the transition from one chemical state to the next, helping this to occur without a massive input of energy. Part of the enzyme enters into a loose chemical combination with one or both of the reactants. It assists in the breaking of existing chemical bonds and in the formation of new ones. Once this process has occurred the enzyme is released, unchanged, and can be re-used. Substances that act in this way are known as **catalysts** (Fig. 2.15).

An enzyme is not consumed in the reaction it catalyses and in theory its concentration will remain unchanged. In practice enzymes slowly deteriorate and must eventually be replaced. In some ways an enzyme is similar to the oil in a car engine which is not burnt as a fuel but eventually has to be renewed (Fig. 2.16).

Almost all the reactions that take place in the body proceed via the aid of a catalyst. A different catalyst is required for each transition. If the reaction proceeds in stages several different enzymes may be involved in one relatively simple process. Some enzymes are known by common names that have been in use for a considerable time. An example is **trypsin**, which is involved in the reactions occurring during the digestion of protein. Others are known by longer names that describe the particular chemical reaction catalysed. During muscular contraction ATP must be combined with part of the myosin component of muscle. The enzyme that catalyses this reaction is known as **myosin ATP-ase**. **Succinate dehydrogenase** is an enzyme that catalyses the removal of hydrogen from succinic acid, a step in the conversion of foodstuffs into carbon dioxide and water. The main processes involved in energy metabolism are summarised in Fig. 2.17 and a few of the important enzymes are listed in Table 2.3. Some enzymes have several different forms or work in conjunction with other substances known as **co-enzymes**. For example, there are several different **iso-enzymes** of lactate dehydro-

Fig. 2.15 Role of the catalyst in a chemical reaction. Without the catalyst the energy a_1 must be input before the reaction can start. This is the activation energy. With a catalyst the activation energy is only a_2.

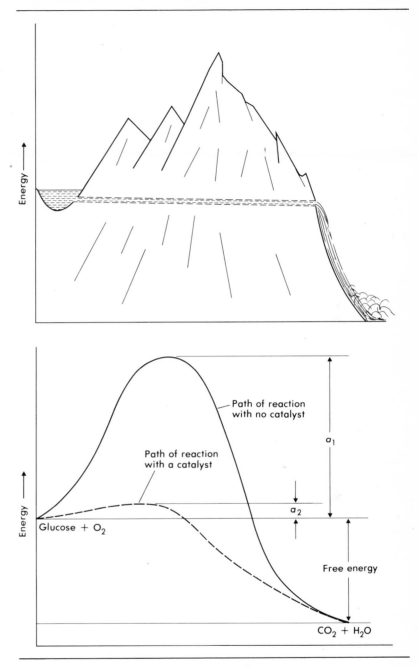

genase. In the discussion which follows all these substances are referred to as *enzymes*.

Figure 2.17 outlines the main processes involved in the breakdown of carbohydrates and fats. Carbohydrates are stored in the liver and skeletal muscle as **glycogen** – an insoluble form of glucose. This is

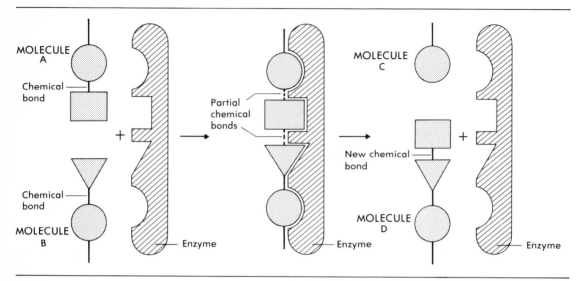

Fig. 2.16 Action of an enzyme catalyst. Molecules A and B enter into a loose chemical combination with specific sites on the enzyme. This disrupts one of the bonds in molecule A and forms a partial bond with part of molecule B. As a result, part of A is transferred to B and two new molecules, C and D, are formed.

Fig. 2.17 Summary of processes involved in the release of energy from carbohydrates and fats.

broken down in several stages until **pyruvic acid** is formed. The process is known as **glycolysis** and results in the formation of a small amount of ATP which can be used for muscular contraction. Several different enzymes are involved in the transition, some of the most important being listed in Table 2.3. Glycolysis normally proceeds in the presence of oxygen (**aerobic metabolism**) when hydrogen is removed from the system with the formation of water. It can also occur in the absence of oxygen (**anaerobic metabolism**). The hydrogen is then used to convert pyruvic acid into lactic acid. This process is catalysed by the enzyme **lactate dehydrogenase** and it allows the production of ATP for muscular contraction under conditions where oxygen is not available. The process has a

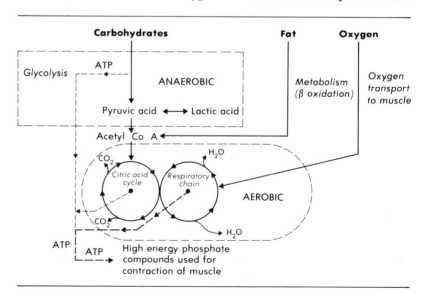

Table 2.3 Names of some enzymes and enzyme-like substances important in muscle and energy metabolism

Name	Common abbreviation	Code	Plays a part in
Glycogen synthase		EC 2.4.1.11	Metabolism of glycogen
Phosphorylase		EC 2.4.1.1	Metabolism of glycogen
Phosphoglucomutase	PGM	EC 2.7.5.1	Metabolism of glycogen
Hexokinase (Phosphohexokinase)	HK PHK	EC 2.7.1.1	Glycolysis
Phosphofructokinase	PFK	EC 2.7.1.11	Glycolysis
Lactate dehydrogenase	LDH or LD	EC 1.1.1.27	Lactic acid metabolism
Citrate synthase	CS	EC 4.1.3.07 EC 4.1.3.28	Citric acid cycle
Succinate dehydrogenase	SDH	EC 1.3.99.1	Citric acid cycle
Malate dehydrogenase	MDH	EC 1.1.1.40	Citric acid cycle
Cytochrome a	Cyt a		Respiratory chain
Cytochrome c	Cyt c		Respiratory chain
Cytochrome oxidase	Cyt ox		Repiratory chain
Lipase	L		Fat metabolism
Alpha-glycerophosphate dehydrogenase	AGPR or AGPD	EC 1.1.1.72	Fat metabolism
Beta-keto-thiolase	BKT	EC 2.3.1.16	Fat metabolism
Acid hydrolase			Protein metabolism
Beta-glucoronidase			Protein metabolism
Carbonic anhydrase		EC 4.2.1.1	Transport of CO_2 in blood
Myosin ATP-ase			Muscular contraction
Ca^{2+} activated ATP-ase	Ca ATP-ase		Muscular contraction
Mg^{2+} activated ATP-ase	Mg ATP-ase		Muscular contraction
Myokinase	MK	EC 2.7.4.3	Muscular contraction
Creatin phosphokinase (Creatin kinase)	CPK CK	EC 2.7.3.2	Muscular contraction

limited capacity, however, because the build-up of lactic acid eventually makes it necessary for the physical activity to be discontinued.

When oxygen *is* available, pyruvic acid is converted into other compounds and metabolised in the **citric acid cycle**, together with the products of fat and protein breakdown. A complex series of reactions occurs resulting in the formation of carbon dioxide. The process is coupled with another series of reactions, known as the **respiratory chain**, in which water is produced. The free energy of each step is slightly lower than that of the preceding one and energy is extracted and used for the formation of ATP. The energy transfer is considerable, producing about eighteen times as much ATP as occurs during glycolysis. A large number of enzymes are involved in the citric acid cycle and respiratory chain. The components of the latter are in fact a series of enzyme-like substances involved in the transfer of energy from the citric acid cycle to ATP. The whole process takes place in microscopic parts of the cell known as **mitochondria**. These are thus responsible for the major part of the energy production in muscle and other kinds of tissue. It has been shown that the capacity to use oxygen is related to the mitochondrial content of muscle, and that both are increased by suitable kinds of endurance training (Barnard *et al.* 1970; Ingjer 1979).

During physical activity ATP is used to provide energy for muscular contraction. Several enzymes take part in this process and in the interconversion of other high-energy phosphate compounds that are also involved.

The rate of a particular chemical reaction is often influenced by the concentration of the principle enzyme involved. This has implications for physical activity because a higher concentration of a key enzyme may allow energy to be produced at a faster rate. The influence of the concentration of the enzymes listed in Table 2.3 on various aspects of physical performance has been investigated. In many cases it has been shown that athletes have a higher concentration of these enzymes than non-athletes. For example, Costill *et al.* (1976a) found that successful runners had about three times the concentration of succinate dehydrogenase in their leg muscles as untrained subjects. This enzyme is involved in the citric acid cycle and an increase in concentration would be expected to benefit performance in middle- and long-distance running. It has also been shown that an increase in enzyme concentrations is one of the effects of training. For example, Thorstensson *et al.* (1975) demonstrated a 36 per cent increase in creatin phosphokinase – an enzyme involved in the release of energy from creatin phosphate – after sprint training.

PARTICULAR ENERGY SOURCES

The various mechanisms by which muscle can obtain energy were shown in Fig. 2.17:(1) from high-energy phosphate compounds; (2) glycolysis; (3) aerobic metabolism of muscle glycogen; and (4) aerobic metabolism of fats and other energy sources. The approximate contribution of each to total power output is illustrated in Fig. 2.18.

An energy source has two important characteristics: the maximum rate at which power can be developed and the duration of its effective operation. It is obvious that an increase in the former will raise the total power output. Figure 2.18 shows that an increase in duration can also have a similar effect. Endurance is thus influenced by both the capacity and maximum power of the various energy sources.

HIGH-ENERGY PHOSPHATE COMPOUNDS

When a muscle contracts and develops force the energy is supplied

Fig. 2.18 Contribution of the various energy sources to total power output. The effect of changing the characteristics of one of the sources is illustrated. Raising either the maximum power output or the duration of operation results in an increase in the total power available.

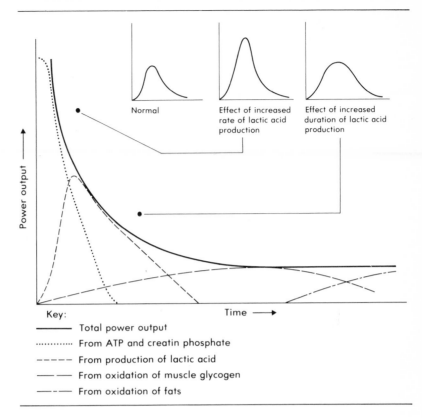

Key:

———— Total power output

············ From ATP and creatin phosphate

– – – – From production of lactic acid

——— From oxidation of muscle glycogen

——·— From oxidation of fats

from the breakdown of adenosine triphosphate (ATP). No other energy source can fulfil this function. ATP consists of an adenosine residue joined to three phosphate groups by relatively high energy bonds. When the last of these is broken its bond energy becomes available for muscular contraction and the molecule is split into two parts: adenosine diphosphate (ADP) and a free phosphate group (P). The reaction can be reversed if energy is available from other sources, such as the metabolism of foodstuffs, and ATP is then manufactured from ADP and P.

The reaction shown in Fig. 2.19 is used as a means of accepting or donating energy. It always occurs in conjunction with a second process that either receives energy from ATP, or provides it, so that ATP is manufactured from ADP and P. ATP is produced during the metabolism of foodstuffs but is used up during the contraction of muscle. In practice these two processes occur simultaneously, ATP acting as a temporary store of energy.

In the resting state aerobic metabolism normally converts almost all muscle ADP and P into ATP. The muscle is effectively provided with an energy store which can be used for contraction irrespective of any other process taking place. The release of energy from ATP is catalysed by enzymes known as **ATP-ases**. It has been shown that the concen-

Fig. 2.19 ATP as a store of energy. Energy is taken in during the breakdown of foodstuffs and released during muscular contraction.

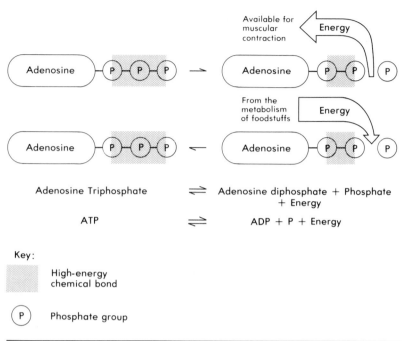

Adenosine Triphosphate $\rightleftharpoons$ Adenosine diphosphate + Phosphate + Energy

ATP $\rightleftharpoons$ ADP + P + Energy

Key:

High-energy chemical bond

(P) Phosphate group

Fig. 2.20 Transfer of chemical energy from glucose to ATP and then from ATP to muscle.

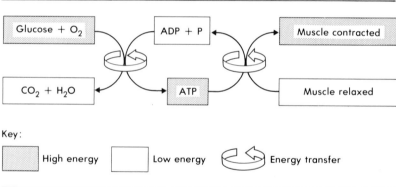

Key:

High energy   Low energy   Energy transfer

tration of these substances is increased by sprint training (Wilkerson and Evonuk 1971; Thorstensson *et al.* 1975). In certain circumstances it is possible to obtain energy from adenosine diphosphate (ADP). Two molecules of ADP combine to form one molecule of ATP which is then used in the normal way. The process is catalysed by the enzyme **myokinase**, the concentration of which is increased by high-intensity training (Thorstensson *et al.* 1975).

2 adenosine diphosphate $\rightarrow$ adenosine monophosphate + adenosine triphosphate

2 ADP $\rightarrow$ AMP + ATP

A further quantity of energy is stored by a second high-energy phosphate compound, **creatin phosphate**. This consists of a combination of creatin and phosphate that can split into these two parts with the release of energy from the chemical bond:

creatin phosphate $\rightleftharpoons$ creatin   +   phosphate   +   energy
CP $\rightleftharpoons$ C   +   P   +   energy

Creatin phosphate is capable of receiving energy only from ATP, and ATP is the only substance its energy can be donated to. It is produced during periods of rest when plenty of energy is available from the metabolism of foods. It is consumed during exercise when ATP is in short supply.

Fig. 2.21 Transfer of chemical energy from ATP to creatin phosphate.

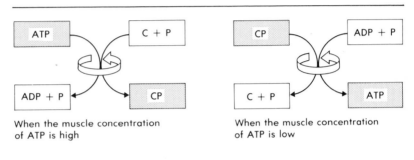

When the muscle concentration of ATP is high

When the muscle concentration of ATP is low

Key: ATP, Adenosine triphosphate;   ADP, Adenosine diphosphate; CP, Creatin phosphate;   C, Creatin;   P, Phosphate

The sole function of creatin phosphate is to act as an extension of the ATP energy store. It is energetically more favourable to employ two different high-energy phosphate compounds rather than a larger amount of ATP. This minimises unfavourable thermodynamic effects which would otherwise reduce the energy available (see Karlson (1968) for details). The roles of ATP and creatin phosphate are summarised in Fig. 2.22.

Of the mechanisms available to the human the high-energy phosphate process provides energy at the highest rate, but it has by far the lowest capacity. The maximum rate of output approaches 100 kcal min^{-1} but at this rate of working the stores are exhausted in only a few seconds. There are variations in both the capacity and power output of the ATP–creatin phosphate system between different individuals and before and after training. A large capacity will allow the individual to work at a relatively high rate for a longer period. It would assist a 200 or 400 m runner because he would be able to complete a greater proportion of the race before having to switch over to other mechanisms that provide energy at a lower rate. However, it would be of more doubtful value to a shot-putter, because the activity is so short. In this case it would be an advantage if the energy from ATP and creatin phosphate could be released at a higher rate.

Training has been shown to affect the concentration of both high-energy phosphate compounds and the enzymes involved in their metab-

Fig. 2.22 Summary of the roles of the various high-energy phosphate compounds.

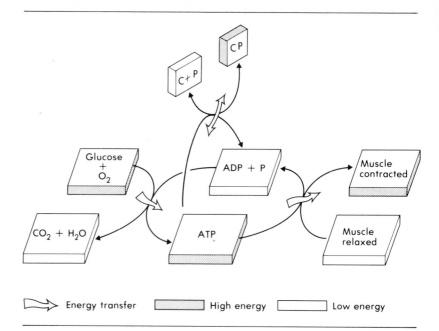

Energy transfer   High energy   Low energy

olism. For example, increases in ATP concentration of 25 and 15 per cent have been reported (Karlsson *et al.* 1972; Houston and Thomson 1977). Some studies have also shown an increase in the creatin phosphate reserves (Eriksson *et al.* 1973) while others report no change (Karlsson *et al.* 1972; Houston and Thomson 1977). Several authors have demonstrated increases in the metabolism of high-energy phosphate compounds (Staudte *et al.* 1973; Thorstensson *et al.* 1975, Costill *et al.* 1979a).

The capacity of the ATP–creatin phosphate system can be expressed in terms of the volume of oxygen needed for the production of an equivalent amount of ATP. Several studies indicate that the effective capacity of the store is equivalent to between 1 and 2 litres of oxygen (Margaria *et al.* 1933; Margaria *et al.* 1964; Roberts and Morton 1978). This energy can be used by muscle in a few seconds – even when working flat out the circulation could not supply oxygen to muscle at this rate. The stores can also be used to supplement the energy obtained aerobically. At the end of a middle-distance race a runner may be pumping 5 litres of oxygen to his muscles each minute. Energy in the ATP–creatin phosphate stores can be used to supplement this during the final burst of speed.

LACTIC ACID SYSTEM – ANAEROBIC GLYCOLYSIS

The lactic acid system is a second method of producing energy under conditions where oxygen is not available. It can provide energy at a faster rate than the aerobic processes and is used during intense activities that last for a minute or so. It is generally brought into operation when the stores of high-energy phosphate compounds are partially exhausted (Margaria *et al.* 1969). It provides energy at a lower rate than the latter process but can be used for a longer period. The capacity of the system is limited by the build-up of lactic acid which prevents further muscular contraction. This has important implications for sport because it may prevent the continuation of physical activity even if adequate energy is available from other sources. In a race lasting about a minute, 70–90 per cent of the energy is obtained from anaerobic processes. Even in events lasting 4 minutes the contribution is 30–40 per cent. After the first few seconds of activity the lactic acid system plays an increasingly important role in the anaerobic production of energy. The successful coach and athlete should be aware of the features of this system and the mechanisms by which it can be developed.

Figure 2.23 illustrates the basis of the lactic acid system and its relationship to the contraction of muscle. All the major components are situated in the muscle cell, close to the contractile filaments, so that the

Fig. 2.23 The metabolism of lactic acid (see text for details).

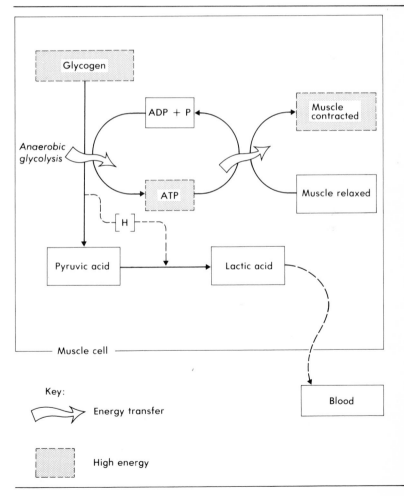

process can occur quickly and without intervention from any other part of the body. Muscle glycogen is converted into pyruvic acid with the manufacture of ATP from ADP and P. This is the process of glycolysis illustrated in Fig. 2.17. The reaction involves the removal of hydrogen from glycogen, and under aerobic conditions this is achieved by combining it with oxygen to produce water. When no oxygen is available the hydrogen is joined to pyruvic acid and lactic acid is formed. This process does not itself release energy but is essential for energy production because without it no glycolysis could occur under anaerobic conditions. Unlike ATP and creatin phosphate, lactic acid is a by-product of a process that produces energy, not the source from which it is obtained. This has important consequences. Although the production of lactic acid indicates that anaerobic glycolysis has occurred, its presence is undesirable because in high concentrations it prevents muscular contraction from taking place. Thus the effectiveness of anaerobic glycolysis as an energy source is influenced by the speed of removal of lactic acid as well as by the rate of production.

Lactic acid production is influenced by several factors including the availability of muscle glycogen. This store of carbohydrate becomes depleted after continuous heavy exercise and the ability to produce lactic acid is then impaired. The capacity for anaerobic glycolysis (production of lactic acid) is improved following certain types of training but the biochemical mechanism by which this occurs is not known with certainty. It is sometimes suggested that an increase in the concentration of **lactate dehydrogenase** – an enzyme involved in the conversion of pyruvic acid to lactic acid – may be responsible. In a recent study Houston and Thomson (1977) have demonstrated an increase in maximum lactic acid production and anaerobic endurance while the concentration of lactate dehydrogenase remained unchanged. This suggests that some other biochemical change is responsible for the improvement. Many other enzymes are involved in anaerobic glycolysis and several authors have shown that the activity of **phosphofructokinase** is increased by training (Eriksson *et al*. 1973; Gollnick *et al*. 1973; Costill *et al*. 1979a). It is possible that this change is responsible for the increased ability to produce lactic acid but a final answer must await further research.

The ability to produce lactic acid is apparently influenced by genetic factors and some investigators suggest that it is not greatly improved by training (Klissouras 1971). It certainly seems more difficult to increase this capacity than many other aspects of fitness (Fox *et al*. 1977; Lesmes 1978b). This may be due to the fact that the enzyme responsible for lactic acid production tends to be located in particular types of muscle fibre and is largely absent from the slow-twitch variety (Costill *et al*. 1976a; Houston and Thomson 1977). Since there are wide individual variations in the percentage of different types of muscle fibre, which appear to be genetically determined, it is perhaps not surprising that the ability to produce lactic acid has a strong genetic component.

Removal of lactic acid The lactic acid produced by muscle finds its way into the bloodstream and is carried round the body. The concentration is easily estimated and is often used as a measure of the energy produced from anaerobic glycolysis. It will be seen later that such scores are sometimes difficult to interpret. The lactic acid content of blood continues to rise for a few minutes after exercise has stopped, due to the time taken for transport from muscle. Blood lactate concentration then slowly declines but may remain elevated for approximately an hour. Until recently this was interpreted as meaning that lactic acid is removed from the body only during recovery from exercise. There is still much controversy about what actually happens to the lactic acid produced in muscle, and the problem is currently receiving a good deal of attention in the scientific literature.

Lactic acid is produced initially because of a lack of oxygen in muscle. As it contains an excess of hydrogen, oxygen is required for its conversion back into more useful substances. It is obvious that the process can occur only in circumstances where oxygen is plentiful – either during recovery, or in parts of the body where oxygen is not in short supply. There are three main possibilities for the removal of lactic acid: (a) conversion back into glycogen or glucose – this requires both oxygen and the input of energy; (b) oxidation to carbon dioxide and water (energy is actually produced during this reaction but its main function is the removal of the toxic lactic acid); and (c) excretion in urine and sweat, which occurs only to a very minor extent (Minaire 1973).

During recovery plenty of oxygen is available in most tissues and the removal of lactic acid is not a particular problem, although it may take a little time. It is very difficult to determine what becomes of lactic acid during recovery, and this may explain why many textbooks and research papers contain such conflicting information. Astrand and Rodahl (1970) state that 85 per cent is converted into glycogen while 15 per cent is oxidised; Mathews and Fox (1976) suggest that 75 per cent is oxidised. The fate of lactic acid probably depends on several factors including the rate of production (Issekutz *et al*. 1976), the level of activity during recovery (Belcastro and Bonen 1975; Stamford *et al*. 1978), the glycogen content of muscle (Piehl 1974; Hermansen and Vaage 1977) and the fibre composition of muscle (Issekutz *et al*. 1976), among others. Hermansen and Vaage (1977) suggest that only a small fraction of the lactate produced during maximal exercise leaves the muscles during recovery and that the major portion may be converted back to glycogen within the muscle. This is a return to a proposal first put forward in 1920 (Meyerhof 1920, 1922).

Lactic acid can also be removed during exercise. The extent to which this process occurs has not been realised until relatively recently. Since the removal of lactate requires oxygen, and its production is a consequence of the lack of oxygen, it follows that lactic acid cannot be removed at the site of production. It must be transported to a place where oxygen is available. Since lactic acid is a carrier of excess hydrogen the

Fig. 2.24 Lactic acid is produced when oxygen is in short supply. Its role is as a carrier of excess hydrogen atoms. During exercise, lactic acid diffuses from the site of production to other parts of the body where it is combined with oxygen. The removal of lactic acid from a muscle cell is thus equivalent to supplying extra oxygen to it.

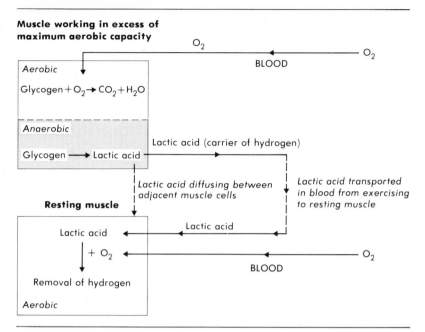

process effectively amounts to a transport of hydrogen away from over-worked muscles to a part of the body where oxygen is plentiful. This process has two important consequences: (1) a greater production of power from anaerobic glycolysis, which occurs because lactic acid is being continually removed so that more can be produced before the concentration reaches a toxic level; and (2) lactic acid can be produced on a continuous basis to supplement the power obtained from aerobic metabolism. The transport of lactic acid *from* a muscle has the same effect as transport of additional oxygen *to* it.

During exercise lactic acid is removed at several times the rate that occurs at rest (Depocas *et al.* 1969; Issekutz *et al.* 1976). The most important sites are skeletal muscle, where it is oxidised to carbon dioxide and water, and the liver, which converts it into glycogen. Between 52 per cent (Depocas *et al.* 1969) and 80 per cent (Minaire 1973) is oxidised by muscle, and the liver appears to account for between 3–4 per cent (Gollnick and Hermansen 1973) and 25 per cent (Issekutz *et al.* 1976). Other tissues, including heart muscle and kidney, are capable of removing small amounts of lactic acid (Keul *et al.* 1972; Nishiitsutsuji-Uwo *et al.* 1967). During exercise there appears to be an increase in blood flow and oxygen uptake in muscle, even in those not directly in-volved in the activity. Muscles switch from the utilisation of fats (the fuel used at rest) to carbohydrates, mainly lactic acid. Ahlborg *et al.* (1975) suggest that 46 per cent of fuel used by resting muscle may con-sist of lactic acid. The ability to remove lactic acid from blood is clearly an advantage to the athlete, but the factors which limit the rate of this process are not known. Jorfeldt *et al.* (1978) found that the mechanism re-

Fig. 2.25 The removal of
lactic acid. An explanation
of the processes is given in
the text.

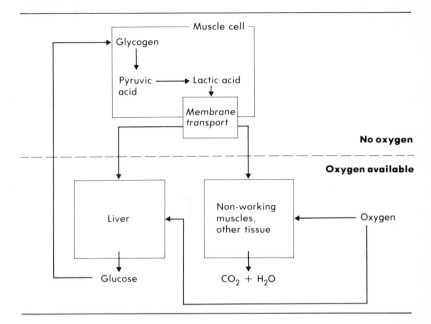

sponsible for transferring lactate from muscle to blood became saturated at high work loads. It is possible that this is the limiting factor.
The removal of lactate during exercise is summarised in Fig. 2.25.

Poortmans *et al.* (1978) have shown that removal of lactate by non-
exercising muscle stops soon after the end of the activity. For this
reason the recovery from an accumulation of lactic acid is slower during
rest than during light or moderate physical activity (Belcastro and
Bonen 1975; Stamford *et al.* 1978). This is one of the reasons why recovery from heavy physical activity is faster if the individual jogs or
'warms down' than if he rests completely. Suitable training can increase
the capacity of the lactic acid system. This results in both an increased
capacity for intensive work and changes in blood lactate concentration.
After a few weeks of such training maximum blood lactate concentrations rise (Eddy *et al.* 1977; Houston and Thomson 1977), which is presumably due to an increased capacity for lactate production. After two
or three months of training maximum blood lactate values tend to fall.
Eddy *et al.* (1977) suggest that this is due to an increase in the capacity
for lactate removal.

The lactic acid system is an important energy source in a wide range
of activities. It plays a significant part in running events between 200
and 1,500 m and in the majority of team games. Yet the type of endurance training undertaken by many sportsmen is unlikely to increase its
efficiency and could even have a detrimental effect. It seems relatively
difficult to increase the capacity for anaerobic glycolysis and the
changes are relatively slow. High-intensity work is necessary and this
needs to be started early in the season; it would seem desirable to make
it a continuous feature of the training programme. Many studies have

shown that slow, long-distance training does not increase the capacity of the lactic acid system. There is now a good deal of evidence that training can alter the enzyme profiles of certain types of muscle fibre. A number of authors have found a decrease in the concentration of glycolytic enzymes following low-intensity endurance training (Baldwin *et al.* 1973; Baldwin *et al.* 1977; Hickson *et al.* 1976; Vihko *et al.* 1979) and a lower concentration in endurance training athletes (Costill *et al.* 1976a, 1976b). The study of muscle biochemistry is in its early stages and the functional significance of these changes remains to be fully investigated. But it would not be surprising if muscle adapted to meet the kind of stress imposed on it, and it seems unwise to place undue emphasis on low-intensity training when a different type of training is likely to be more beneficial.

AEROBIC PRODUCTION OF ENERGY

The aerobic system produces energy by combining carbohydrates, fats and some protein with oxygen. Carbon dioxide and water are formed as by-products. The free energy of the starting materials is transferred to ATP which is used for muscular contraction. This process takes place inside the muscle and it is necessary to transport oxygen there before the reactions can take place. In terms of total energy production this system is by far the most important. It is used exclusively at rest and during moderate forms of continuous activity. It also serves to replenish the other energy systems when they are exhausted. During exercise it is used for activities which last for more than a minute or so. Maximum power is less than with the other two systems but energy can be provided for very much longer. In activities that last more than about 2 minutes it is the capacity of the aerobic system that limits the work output. The system is complex and has a number of separate parts. As a result it is possible to distinguish several components of aerobic endurance which serve to limit performance under different conditions.

The basis of the aerobic production of energy is illustrated in Fig. 2.26. It is clear that the process is more complex than the other methods of energy production, and more than just muscle is involved. The bulk of the energy comes from reactions occurring in the citric acid cycle and respiratory chain. Acetyl CoA and its derivatives are combined with oxygen and for this process to occur there are three principle requirements: a source of fuel (usually acetyl CoA), oxygen, and an adequate concentration of the enzymes of the citric acid cycle and respiratory chain. Any of the three is capable of limiting the amount of energy available from aerobic metabolism and so may affect athletic performance.

The fuel is perhaps the most straightforward of the three requirements. Acetyl CoA, or related compounds, can be produced from any of the three major foodstuffs – carbohydrates, proteins or fats. The production is most rapid when it takes place from the carbohydrate glycogen, which is stored in muscle. There is usually enough for about 1

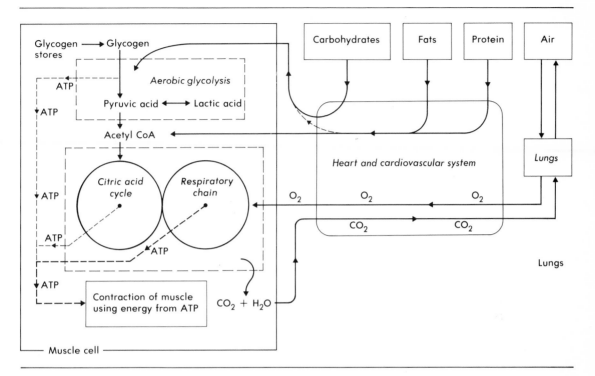

Fig. 2.26 Summary of processes occurring in the aerobic production of energy. The raw materials are oxygen, muscle glycogen, other carbohydrates, fats, and occasionally the breakdown products of protein. All except muscle glycogen must be taken into the muscle cell by the cardiovascular system.

hour or so of heavy physical activity, and as long as adequate muscle glycogen is available energy can be produced at a high rate. As soon as the muscle glycogen stores are depleted other fuel must be taken to the muscle by the bloodstream, and this process limits the rate at which energy can be produced. Small amounts of carbohydrate are available in other parts of the body and derivatives of fats and protein can also be used as fuel. These sources are important at rest and during long periods of light or moderate activity, but they do not allow production of energy at the high rate possible from muscle glycogen. Since we have defined endurance as 'the ability to continue working at the highest possible rate' the availability of glycogen obviously has an influence on endurance.

A supply of oxygen is the other requirement. As long as adequate muscle glycogen is available, oxygen transport limits the rate of energy production from aerobic metabolism. Oxygen must be taken from the air to the part of the muscle where the chemical reactions occur. The process involves several different stages which are summarised in Fig. 2.27.

Air enters the lungs where the oxygen diffuses into the bloodstream and combines loosely with haemoglobin. The blood is then pumped into the arteries by the heart and finally into capillaries which run adjacent to the muscle cells. Oxygen then dissociates itself from haemoglobin and diffuses into individual cells, to the mitochondria, where the

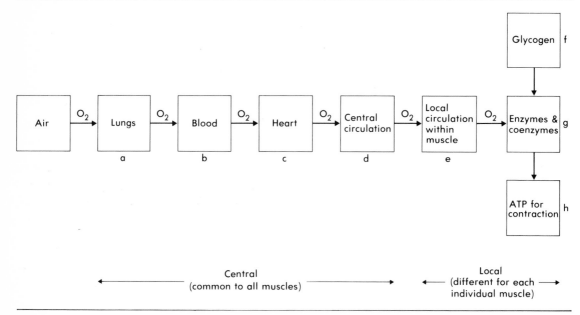

Fig. 2.27 Stages in the aerobic production of ATP for muscular contraction. The efficiency of the process depends on factors peculiar to individual muscles as well as the characteristics of the cardio-respiratory system.

citric acid cycle and respiratory chain are located. Enzymes catalyse the chemical reactions which result in oxygen being used up so that energy can be released. The first four of these stages (a, b, c and d) are centrally located and therefore common to all muscles in the body. The remainder are situated in individual muscles. Aerobic capacity is usually measured in terms of **maximum oxygen uptake**. This is the number of litres of oxygen that the individual can consume in 1 minute of maximum exercise and is often abbreviated to $\dot{V}_{O_2,max}$. Maximum oxygen uptake is influenced by size as well as the efficiency of aerobic processes, so that it is often expressed in terms of the uptake of oxygen per kilogram of body weight. Typical values for various types of athlete are given in Table 2.4.

An individual's maximum oxygen uptake depends partly on the

Table 2.4 Maximum oxygen uptake of untrained individuals and different types of athlete (males)

Subjects	$\dot{V}_{O_2\ max}$ (litre min^{-1})	$\dot{V}_{O_2\ max}$ per kg body weight (ml $kg^{-1}\ min^{-1}$)
Cross-country skiers	5.42	78.3
Long-distance runners	5.19	78.1
Speed skaters	5.58	72.9
800 m runners	5.04	69.8
Cyclists	4.88	67.1
Canoeists	5.25	66.1
Sprinters	4.33	57.1
Untrained	3.14	38.2

Data from Burke *et al.* (1977) and Rusko *et al.* (1978)

capacity of the central cardio-respiratory system and partly on the characteristics of individual muscles. The features of each link in this chain are considered below.

Components of the cardio-respiratory system

The lungs are worked by the respiratory muscles and are responsible for the mixing of air and blood. It is usually accepted that lung function does not limit oxygen transport in normal athletes when working at sea level (Cotes 1965; Shephard 1971). The situation may be different with other types of individual or when work is done at high altitude or under water using breathing aids. Readers requiring further information about exercise under these conditions are referred to the sources above and to Guyton (1966).

The volume and composition of blood have an important influence on aerobic capacity. Oxygen is carried in a loose combination with haemoglobin which is contained in the red blood cells. When the concentration of this pigment falls below the normal level, oxygen transport is reduced in direct proportion to the reduction in haemoglobin concentration. The influence of diet on this factor is discussed later. Haemoglobin concentration may be temporarily reduced soon after the start of a training programme. This occurs because blood volume increases at a faster rate than the production of new red blood cells. Eventually the amount of haemoglobin increases so that its concentration is similar to that at the start of training. The extra blood volume is an advantage because it increases the efficiency of the heart's pumping action. This occurs for two reasons: first, the output of blood per beat is increased; second, the extra volume allows this to be achieved with a lower rate of flow so that less energy is wasted through turbulence (Falch and Strome 1979). Blood volume becomes reduced during dehydration, and this will decrease the efficiency of oxygen transport. The situation is likely to occur during exercise in a hot environment when a great deal of sweating takes place.

The heart and major blood vessels limit the amount of blood that can be pumped round the body each minute. This quantity is known as the **cardiac output** (Q). Maximum cardiac output is influenced by the individual's size, the state of training and the volume of the heart. A non-athletic individual could have a maximum cardiac output of 20 litres of blood per minute while in a well-trained endurance athlete the figure might be as much as 35. A greater cardiac output allows more oxygenated blood to be pumped to the muscles and increases the capacity for the aerobic production of energy. Cardiac output depends upon the number of times the heart beats each minute (*heart rate*) and the volume of blood pumped with each beat (*stroke volume*):

cardiac output = heart rate × stroke volume

Oxygen transport is therefore facilitated if the individual has a high maximum heart rate and a large maximum stroke volume. The high cardiac output of the endurance athlete is due to the latter factor. The maximum stroke volume is likely to be almost 0.2 litre while in the untrained non-athlete it could be only just over 0.1 litre. There are a number of reasons for this difference. Endurance athletes have larger hearts, probably due to genetic factors. Also, their heart muscle is able to develop a great force of contraction so that a greater volume of blood is expelled with each heart beat. This may be partly due to the effects of training on the contraction of heart muscle but it is mainly due to changes in the circulation. Trained individuals have a larger blood volume and a more efficient return of blood to the heart (venous return). This causes a greater stretch of the heart muscle during the filling phase of the cardiac cycle and results in more force being developed when the heart muscle contracts. Contrary to popular opinion, training seems to have little, if any, effect upon the heart size of adults (Ekblom *et al.* 1968; Wolfe *et al.* 1979). The increase in stroke volume is due to the effect described above.

It is often not appreciated that the circulation has an important influence upon stroke volume and cardiac output. The diameter of the arteries and veins is under neural control and this influences both the resistance to blood flow and the rate of return of blood to the heart. This, in turn, affects the degree of stretch of cardiac muscle, and that has an important influence upon stroke volume and cardiac output. The heart is thus the servant of the circulation as well as its master. The relationship between these variables has been extensively investigated by Guyton and his colleagues (Guyton 1963, 1968; Guyton *et al.* 1956). Part of the response to endurance training consists of an increase in blood volume and adaptions in the control mechanisms that regulate blood vessel diameter and blood flow. These changes occur relatively soon after the start of training and are sometimes mistaken for an increase in the size and efficiency of the heart.

In contrast to the situation with stroke volume, there is no clearly established difference between the maximum heart rate of athletes and non-athletes, or trained and untrained individuals. If the maximum heart rate could be raised this would increase cardiac output. But training does not have this effect – it may even cause a slight decrease in maximum heart rate. The literature is not clear on this point. Moffatt *et al.* (1977) quote five studies in which training was found to have no effect upon maximum heart rate and five others in which a slight decrease was observed.

From the arteries the blood travels into capillaries that run inside the body of the muscles, close to individual cells. There is a certain amount of dispute in the scientific literature as to whether endurance training increases the number of capillaries in muscle. Part of the difficulty arises because the older investigations were undertaken using the light microscope which does not distinguish clearly between capillaries and certain other types of tissue. More recent studies, using the electron microscope, confirm that endurance training does increase the ratio of capillaries to muscle fibres (see Ingjer (1979) for details). The widespread belief that low-speed, long-distance running is particularly effective in increasing capillary density has yet to be confirmed by a study employing the electron microscope. At the moment there appears to be no evidence that this type of training is more effective than any other method.

Oxygen diffuses from capillary blood into individual muscle cells where it enters into the chemical reactions that lead to the release of energy. It is only at this point that fuel supply and oxygen finally come into contact. The process takes place in many small steps each of which makes a contribution to the production of ATP. Many different enzymes are involved and the concentration of some of these seems to limit the rate at which the uptake of oxygen can occur. Several recent investigators have found that maximum oxygen uptake is significantly related to the concentration of enzymes of the citric acid cycle and respiratory chain. For example, Costill et $al.$ (1976a) found a correlation of 0.79 between $\dot{V}_{O_2max}$ and the activity of succinate dehydrogenase and Vihko et $al.$ (1978) report that $\dot{V}_{O_2max}$ is related to the activity of several enzymes of the citric acid cycle and respiratory chain. One of the effects of endurance training is to increase the concentration of these enzymes and co-enzymes (Baldwin et $al.$ 1972; Holloszy 1967; Barnard and Peter 1971). This allows greater oxygen utilisation and results in an increase in the individual's maximum oxygen uptake. These studies show that $\dot{V}_{O_2max}$ is influenced just as much by oxygen utilisation inside muscle as by the ability of the cardiovascular system to pump this gas round the body. The chemical events that take place inside the muscle cell actually have an important influence upon the amount of oxygen transported by the blood. This statement may cause surprise because most people see oxygen transport as a process whereby the gas is forcefully pushed into muscle by the lungs and heart, somewhat like the injection of a drug with a hypodermic syringe. In fact the process is closer to the sucking action of a vacuum cleaner. This occurs largely because of the chemical properties of haemoglobin, which are outlined below.

Haemoglobin is the red pigment found in blood. It has the property of being able to combine with oxygen when plenty of this gas is present, but of releasing itself from the combination when oxygen is scarce:

haemoglobin + oxygen $\rightleftarrows$ oxyhaemoglobin
when oxygen is plentiful $\rightarrow$
$\leftarrow$ when oxygen is scarce

The percentage of haemoglobin molecules that are combined with oxygen depends upon the concentration of oxygen in the atmosphere that surrounds the haemoglobin. For example, in the lungs about 98 per cent of all haemoglobin molecules are combined with oxygen. If the concentration of oxygen is reduced to half this value only just over 80 per cent of the haemoglobin remains combined. The relationship is shown graphically in Fig. 2.28.

Fig. 2.28 The oxygen–haemoglobin dissociation curve.

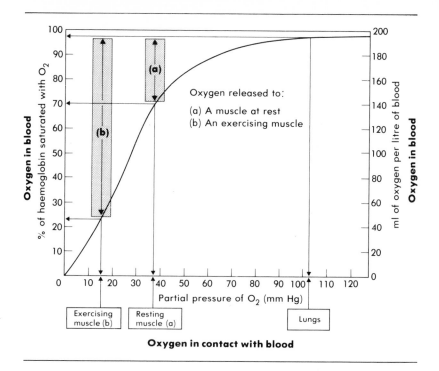

Oxygen released to:

(a) A muscle at rest
(b) An exercising muscle

Oxygen in contact with blood

The concentration of free oxygen is shown along the bottom of the graph. It is expressed as the partial pressure of oxygen, which in the lungs is about 104 mm of mercury. The left-hand axis shows the percentage of haemoglobin molecules that are combined with oxygen. This ranges from about 98 per cent at the partial pressure found in the lungs, down to 0 per cent when the oxygen concentration is zero. The right-hand axis shows the volume of oxygen that is joined to the haemoglobin contained in 1 litre of blood.

Figure 2.28 shows that at the partial pressure of oxygen found in the lungs about 98 per cent of haemoglobin is combined so that 1 litre of blood carries nearly 200 ml of oxygen. If this is transported to a muscle where the partial pressure is between 30 and 40 mm Hg (**a**) only 70 per cent of the haemoglobin remains combined and 18 per cent gives up its oxygen to the muscle. If the muscle is using oxygen rapidly so that the partial pressure is reduced to about 15 mm Hg (**b**) only just over 20 per cent of the haemoglobin remains combined and about 75 per cent gives up its oxygen to the muscle. The amount of oxygen delivered by the blood thus depends upon the demands of the tissue. One litre of blood supplies about 50 ml of oxygen to muscle **a** while to **b** the same blood donates nearly 150 ml. When the blood is returned to the lungs the haemoglobin once again becomes 98 per cent saturated so that it again contains about 200 ml of oxygen per litre. The process requires the passage of oxygen from the lungs into the bloodstream. A litre of blood returned from muscle **a** will absorb 50 ml of oxygen while the

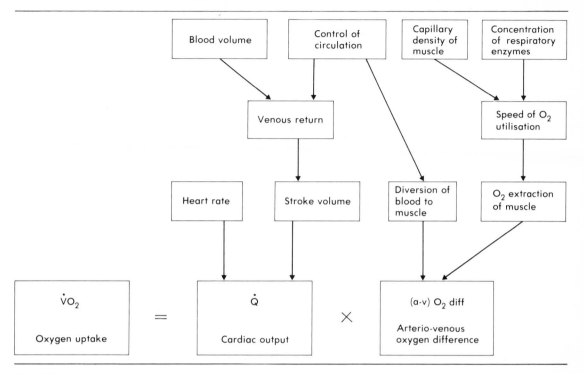

Fig. 2.29 Factors which influence cardiac output, (a-v) O_2 difference and thus $\dot{V}_{O_2max}$.

same volume of blood from muscle **b** will take in 150 ml. This example makes it clear that the metabolism of muscle not only controls the release of oxygen from blood but also influences the amount that is taken into the bloodstream in the lungs.

During exercise three additional factors increase the transfer of oxygen from haemoglobin to muscle: raised muscle temperature, acidity due to carbon dioxide production, and the presence of 2,3-diglycerophosphate – a compound involved in the metabolism of carbohydrates. These three factors facilitate the release of oxygen from haemoglobin making more of the gas available to muscle. Ramsey and Pipoly (1979) have shown that lactic acid reduces 2,3-diglycerophosphate concentration. This has the effect of reducing the capacity of the aerobic system and may be a problem in poorly trained individuals who produce lactic acid at low levels of energy expenditure.

It should now be clear that the volume of oxygen delivered to muscle is influenced by the amount removed from blood as well as by the rate of blood flow. The volume of oxygen removed from blood is the difference between the volume that is contained in 1 litre of arterial blood and the volume returned to the lungs in the veins. This quantity is known as the arterio-venous oxygen difference, (a-v)O_2 diff. For example, in Fig. 2.28 the following applies to the blood flow to muscle (a):

Oxygen in 1 litre of arterial blood	*Oxygen in 1 litre of venous blood*	*Oxygen removed from 1 litre of blood*
180 ml	140 ml	40 ml

47

Thus the (a-v)O_2 difference is 40 ml O_2 per litre of blood.

When a muscle is working hard it can remove almost all the oxygen from the blood supplied to it. However, not all blood flow goes to working muscle, some is directed to tissues which extract little oxygen. The average (a-v)O_2 difference for the whole body depends upon how effectively blood can be diverted to the muscles that are active. There are several physiological mechanisms which help achieve this (for details see Guyton (1966), and their effectiveness is probably increased by training. A well-trained endurance athlete can extract the major portion of the oxygen contained in arterial blood, his (a-v)O_2 difference being over 150 ml of oxygen per litre of blood.

In an earlier section we saw that the capacity for the aerobic production of energy is measured as the individual's maximum oxygen uptake. It should now be clear that this is determined both by the rate of blood flow (cardiac output) and the degree of oxygen extraction (arterio-venous oxygen difference):

oxygen uptake $=$ rate of blood flow $\times$ degree of oxygen removal from blood (arterio-venous oxygen difference)

$$\dot{V}_{O_2} \quad = \quad \dot{Q} \quad \times \quad (a\text{-}v)O_2 \text{ diff.}$$

A high maximum oxygen uptake will result from a high cardiac output and a large (a-v)O_2 difference. Some of the factors which influence these two variables are shown in Fig. 2.29. Several recent studies confirm that the ability to transport oxygen is influenced by the characteristics of muscle as well as by the action of the heart. Muscles that have undergone endurance training can extract more oxygen from blood than others. Thus rowers attain a greater maximum oxygen uptake while rowing than when they run on a treadmill; cyclists have a higher $\dot{V}_{O_2 max}$ while cycling than when running or undertaking any other kind of activity. It has also been shown that training has a specific effect on oxygen uptake. Swim-training increases the maximum oxygen uptake when swimming but not during running; run-training has a greater effect on the $\dot{V}_{O_2 max}$ measured during running than on the $\dot{V}_{O_2 max}$ measured during swimming. These studies are considered in more detail in the section on endurance training in Chapter 4.

LONG-TERM ENDURANCE

Some sports involve a prolonged period of physical activity – long-distance running, canoeing, skiing and cycling are examples. In such activities endurance can be influence by one or more of a large number of different factors. The more important include: the supply of nutrients, cardiovascular function, the ability to regulate body temperature, water and electrolyte loss, tissue breakdown and injury, resistance to fatigue. Each of these is considered briefly below.

Fuel supply During prolonged physical activity the stores of muscle glycogen become exhausted and energy is obtained from other fuels supplied via the bloodstream. These include glucose obtained from glycogen that is stored in the liver, fats, and chemicals derived from the breakdown of protein. The release of these substances is controlled by a complex series of hormones that match the supply of fuel to the demands of the muscles. The system is not yet fully understood but it appears that training leads to changes in the hormonal balance during exercise (Hickson *et al.* 1979). Diet has an important influence on the availability of fuels and this is considered in the section on nutrition.

Cardiovascular function During prolonged exercise there is a gradual decline in the subject's stroke volume and a corresponding increase in heart rate (Saltin and Stenberg 1964; Rowell 1974). It is not known for certain whether this is due to fatigue of the heart muscle, or to other causes. Maher *et al.* (1978) suggest that it is probably due to changes occurring in the circulation which lead to a pooling of blood and a decrease in the venous return to the heart.

Temperature regulation Physical activity leads to a massive generation of heat. When working hard an athlete produces about as much heat as a one-bar electric fire. If steps were not taken to secure the removal of this heat a fatal rise in body temperature would rapidly occur. One of the constraints upon long-term endurance is the ability to maintain body temperature at a normal level.

There are two principle mechanisms for heat loss. Large quantities of blood are diverted to the skin where energy is lost from the body by convection, conduction and radiation. This process requires the diversion of blood away from the working muscles so that their oxygen supply is reduced. This results in a corresponding drop in work output. The other mechanism involves the production of sweat which evaporates, taking heat away from the body. The latter process is more efficient in that it involves the diversion of less blood away from working muscle. Endurance training appears to reduce the temperature at which sweating begins so that more of the cardiac output is reserved for the transport of oxygen to the tissues (Gisolfi 1973; Henane *et al.* 1977; Nadel 1979). A similar but more pronounced effect occurs in the process of acclimatisation to a hot environment (Wyndham 1967). Sweat consists of water and certain salts. These are obtained from plasma, the watery part of blood. Thus sweating results in a reduction in blood volume and a loss of electrolytes from the body. If much water is lost, venous return and cardiac output are compromised and the blood supply to muscle is reduced. When the subject becomes dehydrated sweating is reduced and eventually stops altogether. Body temperature then rises and the individual succumbs to heat stroke. There is an increased risk of heat stroke in children and old people (Drinkwater and Horvath 1979). During long periods of activity fluid losses should be replaced as they occur and the athlete obviously should not begin the activity in a state of partial dehydration. Other ways in which the athlete can minimise the problem of heat dissipation are through endurance training, acclimatisation to heat, and wearing the minimum of clothing appropriate to the activity; natural fibres generally allow for better evaporation of sweat. When the relative humidity is high, the evaporation of sweat is reduced. If the environmental temperature is also high heat cannot be lost from the body by conduction or convection and any form of prolonged activity will inevitably lead to heat stroke. For further information on temperature regulation the reader is referred to the following sources: Mathews and Fox (1976), Wyndham (1973) and Nadel (1977).

Prolonged exercise may also be limited by several other factors. Fatigue in the nervous system is a likely candidate. This is not meant to imply that the individual simply stops trying. Changes in the function of the nervous system may prevent the activity being continued or indicate that it must take place at a considerably reduced rate (Asmussen and Mazin 1978).

It is likely that tissue damage also has an important effect. Enzymes and other chemicals leak from muscle, and this may be responsible for a decline in power output with time. Strenuous exercise can increase the urinary excretion of protein up to one hundred times (Poortmans and Jeanloz 1978); some of this may be due to simple leakage, but there is evidence that tissue breakdown also occurs (Williams and Ward 1977). The various mechanisms concerned with energy production are summarised in Fig. 2.30.

SPEED

The term 'speed' is applied to a variety of different phenomena that occur in sport: fast reactions, a burst of rapid movement, the ability to run continuously at high speed. **Reaction time** is a property of the nervous system and depends upon the speed at which information is processed. A burst of rapid movement involves the translation of reaction into motion. It requires acceleration of the body, or part of it, and the continuation of movement at high speed.

In mechanical terms, speed is the distance covered in a given time:

$$\text{speed} = \frac{\text{distance}}{\text{time}}$$

It is measured in terms of distance per unit time, for example: miles per hour (mph); feet per second (ft s^{-1}); metres per second (m s^{-1}).

Acceleration specifies how rapidly speed is changed. A car that can go from rest to 60 mph in 20 seconds has greater acceleration than one that takes 60 seconds. Acceleration is thus speed/time:

$$\text{acceleration} = \frac{\text{speed}}{\text{time}} = \frac{\text{distance}}{\text{time}} \times \frac{1}{\text{time}} = \frac{\text{distance}}{(\text{time})^2}$$

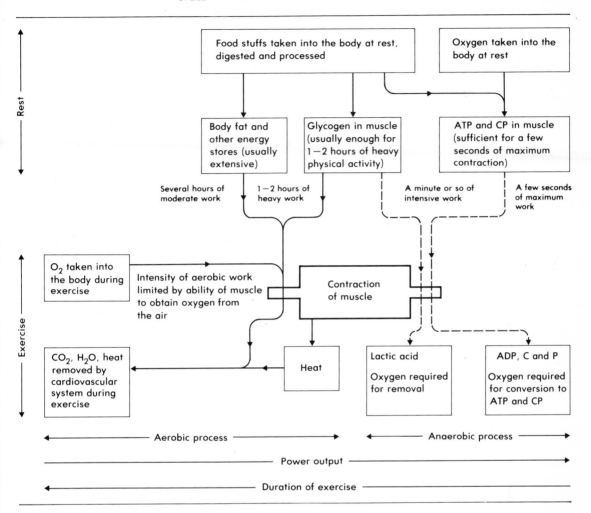

Going from left to right, the activity becomes

| | | |

Fig. 2.30 Summary of energy metabolism during exercise of different intensities. The top half of the diagram illustrates processes occurring at rest; the lower half shows those taking place during exercise. Going from left to right, the activity becomes shorter but of greater intensity.

Acceleration is measured in terms of distance per second squared, for example: metres per second squared ($m\ s^{-2}$); feet per second squared ($ft\ s^{-2}$). For example, the acceleration due to the earth's gravitational field is approximately $9.75\ m\ s^{-2}$. Consider the case of a runner who starts at rest and accelerates at a rate of $3\ m\ s^{-2}$. After 1 second his speed will be $3\ m\ s^{-1}$. During the course of the next second his speed will again increase by $3\ m\ s^{-1}$ so that at the end of 2 seconds the runner's speed will be $6\ m\ s^{-1}$. After 5 seconds the speed will be $15\ m\ s^{-1}$.

Acceleration does not occur unless a force is applied to an object. In the case of a runner this is provided mainly by the muscles of the legs. The amount of acceleration is influenced both by the mass of the body and the force applied to it. The relationship is specified in Newton's second law of motion which can be stated as:

$$\text{acceleration} = \frac{\text{force}}{\text{mass}}$$

Fig. 2.31 The relationship between acceleration, speed and distance covered. (a) Acceleration occurs at 3 m s^{-2} for 5 s and then drops to zero. (b) After 5 s the speed is 15 m s^{-1} and then remains constant. (c) After 5 s the distance covered is about 38 m; 112 m after 10 s.

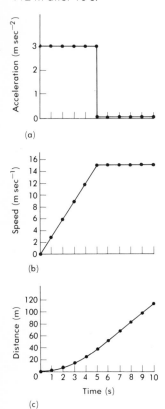

(a)

(b)

(c)

Time (s)

The acceleration will be doubled if the force causing it is doubled, but is halved if the mass of the object increases two-fold. In sporting situations acceleration will be improved by increasing the force available from muscular contraction and by reducing the weight of the object to be moved.

In throwing events the weight of the projectile is fixed and acceleration can be improved only by applying greater force. In running, jumping and all other activities involving movement of the body there is generally some room for weight reduction through the removal of non-essential tissue such as fat. The gains in acceleration will be proportional to the decrease in body weight. Sprinters should not be tempted to lose weight by becoming dehydrated. This will have an adverse effect on the ability to develop force. The force available for acceleration is not usually the same as that developed by the muscles. Losses due to joint friction and tissue viscosity must be subtracted. In some individuals excess fat in the arms and thighs makes these limbs 'tight' and results in considerable loss of muscular force. It is difficult to measure this effect and, as far as is known, it has never been systematically studied. In the author's view, limb-tightness does have an adverse effect upon performance.

The force–velocity relationship of muscle is also relevant to acceleration. It was shown earlier that the force developed by a muscle depends upon its speed of contraction. A high level of static strength will assist the athlete in the initial phase of motion. But if the acceleration is to be maintained, it is also necessary that adequate force is developed when the speed of contraction is high (for further details see the section on strength earlier in this chapter).

In running there is no clear-cut distinction between acceleration and moving at constant velocity. Once top speed has been reached it is still necessary to accelerate the limbs, which are stationary twice in each cycle of movement. Considerable energy expenditure is also required to move the body up and down and to overcome tissue and air resistance.

The ability to run at high speed is, to a large extent, a matter of skill, and much of this is inherited rather than acquired. Improvements in speed are possible through training but tend to be smaller than the

Table 2.5 Places on school and county teams (athletics excluded) of juveniles attending an athletics coaching course in Norwich, 1972

Type of athlete	Number of Subjects	Membership of school teams (places per athlete)*	Membership of county teams (places per athlete)*
Sprinters	20	3.5	0.5
		2–8	0–3
Middle- and long-distance runners	15	1.5	0
		0–4	0–0
Field athletes	16	2.1	0.2
		1–5	0–2

* Mean and range of scores.

gains common with many other aspects of fitness. Sprinting speed is apparently a great advantage in team games and children who are able to sprint well tend to be more successful in gaining places on representative teams.

POWER

Power is about the rate at which work can be done. In athletic situations it is closely related to the development of strength and speed. In physical terms, work is done when an object is moved against the resistance of an opposing force:

work = force × distance

It is easy to calculate the work done when an object is moved through a vertical distance because the motion is opposed by gravity. If a 200 lb man steps onto a chair 1.5 ft high the work done is 200 × 1.5 ft lb, or 300 ft lb. On the metric system work is often measured in kp m. The above action would involve moving 90.91 kg through 0.4572 m and be equivalent to 41.56 kp m of work. These calculations are of the useful work done. Some work is wasted in overcoming tissue and joint resistance. In activities like running there is usually no overall vertical movement although oscillations occur during each stride. These contribute to the work done; so does motion against air and tissue resistance. These factors make it impossible to make a direct calculation of work output, except during vertical movement when the useful work is large compared to that wasted.

Power output can be optimised by reducing some of the wasted force. Well-designed footwear and other equipment will increase traction and allow more force to be usefully applied. Tissue resistance and extraneous weight should be reduced to a minimum. Maximum power output is increased when muscle temperature is raised (Binkhorst et al. 1977).

Power is the amount of work done in unit time. Therefore:

$$\text{power} = \frac{\text{work}}{\text{time}} = \frac{\text{force} \times \text{distance}}{\text{time}}$$

Since speed is distance/time, power is also equal to force × speed.

In the section on strength it was shown that the force developed by a muscle depends upon the speed of contraction. This means that the power output also depends upon speed. This is illustrated in Fig. 2.32. Since power = force × speed, power is zero when either the speed of contraction is zero (an isometric contraction) or the force developed is zero. These are the conditions at the extreme left and right of each graph. Power output rises at intermediate combinations of force and speed and reaches a maximum at about one-third of the maximum speed. In the human, neural mechanisms limit the force developed

Fig. 2.32 *Top*: force and power output for an isolated muscle. *Bottom*: the situation for a muscle in position in the body before and after warm-up.

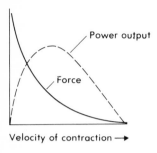

Velocity of contraction →

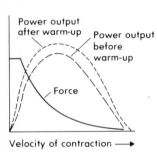

Velocity of contraction →

at low speeds and this results in a corresponding decrease in power output.

Maximum power can be developed for only a few seconds because the energy stores in muscle are rapidly depleted and other, less efficient, sources must then be employed. Intensive exercise increases the size of these stores so that high power output can be maintained for a longer period. This is considered in more detail in the section on endurance.

The so-called *power events* are activities such as jumps, sprints and throwing events. They consist of activities where the athlete's body is propelled – jumping and sprinting – or an external object is projected – a hammer or shot. In the latter type of activity a high body weight is an advantage, provided it is also accompanied by dynamic strength and speed. This is because the momentum of the body can be transferred to the projectile. Weight is not an advantage in sprinting because the body is the object which must be accelerated.

PHYSIQUE

The physique of an individual at a given point in time is known as his phenotype. This is strongly influenced by genetic factors (the genotype) but a certain degree of modification *is* possible.

Physique can be quantified by means of anthropometric measurements – lengths, widths, thicknesses and circumferences of various parts of the body. A large number of such measurements is possible but these can be arranged into groups using a technique known as factor analysis. In one such analysis of 46 measurements taken on 106 sportsmen by the author, three primary factors were obtained. These could each be split into two subfactors corresponding approximately to: upper body muscle, lower body muscle; bone lengths, bone widths; and two fat factors. There were considerable variations in the magnitude of these six factors between different types of sportsmen.

BONE SIZES

These determine the basic size and shape of the individual and are capable of little, if any, modification. It is possible that prolonged training may result in a slight thickening of bone but there is no evidence that exercise has any effect on bone length.

MUSCLE CIRCUMFERENCES

Muscle girths can be modified by training within certain limits. These are probably determined by somatotype and other genetically fixed characteristics. The relationship between the size of individual muscles and individual bones is often only slight; but taken in combination muscle girths do seem to be significantly related to bone lengths and widths. In the study quoted above it was found that 75.5 per cent of the

Fig. 2.33 *Top*: much of the stability of the knee joint is derived from the strength of muscles which run from the pelvis to the bones of the leg. *Bottom*: well-developed muscles round the knee joint and the type of situation in which the knee is likely to give way.

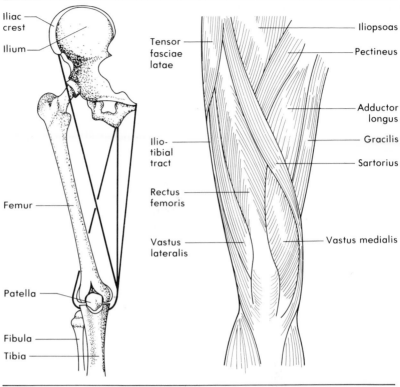

Iliac crest

Ilium

Tensor fasciae latae

Iliopsoas

Pectineus

Ilio-tibial tract

Adductor longus

Gracilis

Sartorius

Femur

Rectus femoris

Vastus lateralis

Vastus medialis

Patella

Fibula

Tibia

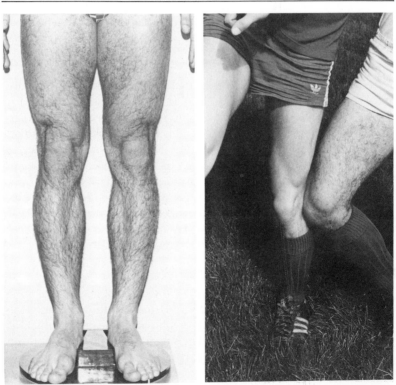

variance of the muscle circumferences of 106 sportsmen could be accounted for by 14 skeletal measurements. This suggests that bone sizes have a much more important influence than training on muscle girths.

In addition to its responsibility for the development of strength, muscle plays a part in the protection of the skeleton from external violence – it acts as an effective form of padding – and assists in the stabilisation of joints. In the knee joint in particular, muscle has an important role in providing lateral stability (Goldfuss *et al.* 1973). Both these aspects of muscle function are important in activities where there is heavy body contact. In a study of schoolboy rugby players it was found that the incidence of injury was related to poor muscle development (Watson 1982).

The balance between muscle groups is also important in avoiding strains and other injuries. Burkett (1970) found that the incidence of hamstring strains was considerably increased if there was muscle imbalance between the two legs. It was also increased if the flexion–extension strength ratio (knee flexor strength/knee extensor strength) deviated from 0.6. A 10 per cent deviation was found to be critical. Imbalance between other muscle groups can lead to postural deviations which may predispose the individual to injury (see section on Posture, opposite).

The sportsman needs sufficient muscle to provide strength, stability and protection, but amounts in excess of this can be a handicap because energy expenditure increases with body weight. Endurance athletes do not generally require great strength and most successful middle- and long-distance runners have relatively little muscle.

FAT

This is used by the muscles as a fuel during light and moderate activity but not usually during strenuous work. It insulates the body against cold and helps prevent hypothermia (exposure). Its chief disadvantage is that it adds non-productive weight to the body. This increases energy expenditure and reduces the ability to accelerate. Excessive fat on the legs seems to reduce anaerobic power output (Watson 1983). Fat also has an adverse effect on dissipation of the heat produced during strenuous activity (Haymers *et al.* 1975). Obese individuals find it more difficult to work in a hot environment (Bar-Or *et al.* 1969; McCormac and Buskirk 1974) and have a greater susceptibility to heat stroke (Schickele, 1947; Minard *et al.* 1957).

BODY WEIGHT

Weight is influenced by the mass of all the individual body tissues and as such is far too general a measure to give much information about physical condition. The components likely to show the greatest fluctuations are water, fat and muscle but the weighing machine does not distinguish between any of these. Even weight *changes* are not particularly informative because a loss in one tissue may be masked by a gain in another.

Following a single session of intensive exercise body weight drops, due almost entirely to water loss through sweating. Significant dehydration is dangerous, being likely to lead to heat stroke; mild dehydration degrades performance by reducing blood volume and upsetting water–electrolyte balance. After exercise the water is quickly replaced; saunas and sticky games of squash do not result in a lasting reduction in body weight.

Following a few days of exercise the body weight usually rises. This is due mainly to retention of water. During longer periods of activity weight is reduced in some individuals through loss of fat. In a group who exercised for one month Watson (1973) found that subjects who began with little fat gained weight, while those who were fat at the start of training lost weight because their fat loss was greater than their gain in non-fat tissue.

POSTURE

Posture is a difficult concept to define. It is really about the alignment of different segments of the body; the spatial relationship of the various portions of the limbs and trunk; their position with respect to the head and feet. Misalignment of some or all of these segments results in postural deviations such as abnormal curvature of the spine or limbs. The term 'body mechanics' is sometimes used with the same meaning. Postural deviations may be due to defects of bones or joints; or they can be caused by inadequate or uneven development of muscle. Abducted or 'winged' scapulae occur when the rhomboids and serratus anterior muscles are weak, allowing the tips of the shoulder blades to protrude at the back, at the same time causing the shoulders to become hunched forward (Fig. 2.34). The condition is exaggerated if in the same individual the muscles which attach to the front of the scapulae are well developed and strong. Other postural defects can be due to similar causes. They include: lumbar lordosis, an exaggerated inward curve of the back in the lumbar region; scoliosis, a sideways curvature of the spine; and dropped foot arches (flat feet). These conditions are illustrated in Fig. 5.19 on p. 169.

The whole area of posture is fraught with difficulties for the investigator. There is no real agreement on what constitutes satisfactory posture, hence assessment is a problem. And many defects have a large number of possible causes making it very difficult to establish relationships. Many writers on the topic believe that certain postural deviations predispose to sports injury but it is difficult to be certain. The present author has reasonable evidence that lumbar lordosis is associated with groin strain due to tightness of the iliopsoas muscle (Watson 1974, and unpublished), and that injury is more common in sportsmen with

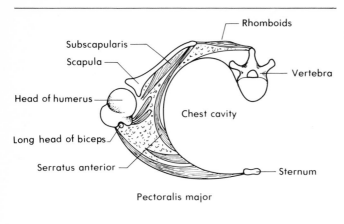

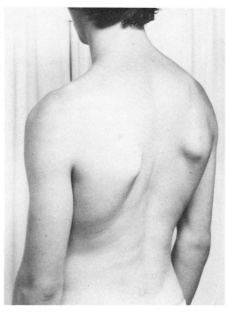

Fig. 2.34 *Left*: cross-section through the trunk at the level of the shoulder. *Right*: abducted scapulae due to weakness of the muscles illustrated in the left-hand diagram.

postural defects. An undergraduate thesis carried out under the author's supervision supports this idea. It also seems possible that excessive specialisation in one particular activity can lead to the development of postural deviations (Watson, unpublished). Kicking, leg lifts and straight leg sit-ups may be associated with lordosis, push-ups and activities which develop the muscles of the anterior trunk with abducted scapulae and asymmetric activities, like many stick or racquet games, with the development of scoliosis.

NUTRITION; FLUID AND ELECTROLYTE BALANCE

FOOD INTAKE

Diet provides the raw materials necessary for energy production. It is also the source of chemicals used in the manufacture and replenishment of structural components of the body, and the various biochemical pathways.

Along with water the principal components of diet are proteins, carbohydrates and fats but several accessory food factors – vitamins and minerals – are also necessary, bringing the total number of essential dietary constituents to around 40. A deficiency of any one of these can have noticeable effects. Proper diet is particularly important for sportsmen, because a high level of physical activity increases the turnover of such substances as proteins and minerals. Exercise frequently results in the leakage or degradation of enzymes in muscle and other tissues and of red blood cells. Damage to connective tissue is also common. Sportsmen must therefore ensure an adequate intake of the precursors of these items, notably protein, iron and other minerals, and certain vitamins. The nutritional requirements of the athlete are complex, and space permits only a few general comments to be made.

Protein

Protein is the source of amino acids from which the body constructs new protein. Animal protein from lean meat, poultry and fish contains all the essential amino acids required by the body. Protein from vegetable sources may lack one or more essential amino acid or contain these substances in the wrong proportions. Although the daily requirements for protein are not high – probably about 1 g of animal protein per kilogram of body weight (Recommended Dietary Allowances, 1968) deficiencies amongst athletes do occur. In an unpublished study the author found that about one-quarter of a group of young athletes had a protein intake which was either inadequate or borderline. This may be partly because foods containing protein tend to be expensive while the financial resources of the young sportsmen are often limited. A second reason is the relatively low proportion of protein contained in foods like meat. Grilled steak contains only 17 per cent protein and the values for the majority of other meat and fish items ranges from 10 to 20 per cent.

Fats and carbohydrates

Fats and carbohydrates are widely distributed in food. Both occur in adequate quantities in most western diets. Carbohydrate intake is of interest because of its influence upon the concentration of glycogen in skeletal muscle. Glycogen is used almost exclusively by muscle during heavy physical activity. After 40–90 minutes of such exercise muscle glycogen stores are exhausted and the muscle is no longer capable of performing heavy work. It has been demonstrated that heavy physical activity can be continued for a longer period if the concentration of glycogen in muscle is high (Bergstrom et al. 1967). This situation can be achieved by a special dietary procedure (Hultman and Bergstrom 1967; Karlsson and Saltin 1971). The individual first empties his muscles of glycogen by an hour or so of heavy physical activity. For the next three days he consumes a diet containing no carbohydrate. This is followed by three days on an almost exclusively carbohydrate diet which contains no protein or fat. The regimen is capable of increasing muscle glycogen stores two- or three-fold. Although there may occasionally be undesirable side-effects the procedure may be of considerable benefit to sportsmen undertaking strenuous events which last for more than an hour or so.

It is well known that the assimilation of carbohydrates leads to a release of the hormone insulin. This in turn tends to inhibit the utilisation of muscle glycogen. Foster et al (1979) have shown that the ingestion of glucose within 30 minutes of heavy physical activity actually leads to a decrease in endurance due to this mechanism. Carbohydrates should therefore be avoided prior to, and at the start of, heavy physical activity.

Vitamins and minerals

Vitamins are required only in minute amounts, although they are essential for normal body function. Most appear to act as co-enzymes in various metabolic processes. A number of the B group vitamins act in this way in the citric acid cycle and respiratory chain. The intake of B group vitamins should be related to energy expenditure. Vitamin C is required for the manufacture of collagen, an important component of connective tissue. It is also involved in the production of red blood cells along with iron, folic acid and vitamin B_{12} (Marks 1968). In a recent study on young sportsmen (Watson and Sheehan unpublished) the incidence of mild anaemia was found to be 34 per cent and was associated with inadequate intake of a number of these accessory food factors. In the author's experience such dietary deficiencies in sportsmen are far from uncommon. However, excessive quantities of vitamins serve no purpose and are simply excreted from the body.

It is sometimes claimed that vitamin E is especially beneficial to athletes. This substance has a function in the muscle metabolism of some animals (Nafstat and Tollersrud 1970) but no role has ever been established for it in man (Helgheim et al. 1979). Although some early investigators have suggested that vitamin E improves performance during exercise of long duration, most recent studies have failed to confirm such claims (Shephard et al. 1974; Watt et al. 1974; Lawrence et al. 1975; Sharman et al. 1976).

WATER AND ELECTROLYTES

Water does not undergo chemical breakdown in the body but a certain amount must be excreted each day in order to remove harmful waste products. Water is also lost during respiration and sweating. Insensible perspiration occurs at all times. During exercise in a hot environment the water loss is considerable and can amount to one gallon, or more, per hour.

Water balance is controlled by osmoreceptors situated in the brain. When water is lost the body fluids become more concentrated. This is detected by the osmoreceptors: a sensation of thirst is produced and the water excretion of the kidney is reduced. The opposite occurs if excessive water is ingested and it is soon excreted as urine. This mechanism normally maintains water balance in man. It is inadequate only when sweating is excessive. The sensation of thirst may then be delayed and dehydration can result. This is a serious situation for two reasons: blood volume is reduced leading to a fall in stroke volume and reduced efficiency of the heart; sweating then stops, in order to conserve blood volume, and the athlete succumbs to heat stroke.

Endurance athletes, and those who exercise in the heat, must ensure an adequate fluid intake. Water losses should be replaced during long races and other forms of prolonged exercise. Drinks are passed from the stomach to the small intestine more rapidly if they are cool (Costill and Saltin 1974). The presence of glucose and other sugars retards this process. Costill and Saltin have demonstrated that 60–70 per cent of a 400 ml draft of water leaves the stomach in 15 minutes while only 5 per cent of a drink containing 10 per cent sucrose leaves in the same time. The assimilation of strong solutions of sugar is very slow. For rapid absorption drinks should contain not more than 2.5 per cent of carbohydrates. The presence of electrolytes also retards the passage of fluids from the stomach and any strong solution is unsuitable for the rapid replacement of water losses. Large quantities of fluid take some time to leave the stomach whatever their composition, and fluid-replacement drinks should be limited to volumes of 100–200 ml (3 to 6 oz). In extreme conditions such replacement may be needed at 10–15 minute intervals. An intake of 500 ml of fluid (approximately 15 oz) may be useful about 30 minutes before the start of a long event: earlier ingestion will result in its conversion to urine. Such a drink should not contain significant quantities of carbohydrates or the mobilisation of muscle glycogen reserves may be impaired.

It is well known that sweat contains electrolytes in addition to water. However, the concentration of sodium and chloride in sweat is only about one-third that of plasma, so that relatively more water is lost than salt and sweating leaves the body fluids more concentrated. Water is required to restore the balance and the ingestion of salt actually makes the situation worse. Costill (1977a) has questioned the value of athletic drinks which contain electrolytes such as sodium, chloride, potassium and magnesium, the body's immediate need being water. He suggests that electrolytes should be replaced after exercise by drinking a glass of orange or tomato juice and by adding a little more salt to the diet. Costill has produced an excellent review of the use of fluids during exercise, and it is recommended for those requiring further information (Costill 1977a).

Lack of mineral intake may occasionally lead to bouts of cramp, although there are also a number of other causes of this disorder. Athletes suffering from bouts of cramp should try a little more salt with their food.

Dehydration is occasionally a progressive phenomenon. Changes in body weight are a reasonable guide to water loss and athletes should keep an accurate daily record of their weight. This should be measured in the morning, after urinating but before eating or drinking.

HEALTH

MAINTAINING THE SPORTSMAN IN TOP PHYSICAL CONDITION

The well-trained athlete is similar to a highly tuned racing car in which the slightest mechanical malfunction is likely to cause a noticeable reduction in performance or lead to breakdown during the stress of competition. In an 'old banger' quite serious defects often pass unnoticed. This is because they are masked by other problems and because the demands made on the vehicle are of a much lower order. In the athlete minor malfunctions can have serious, even devastating, consequences. For example, a slight degree of anaemia will negate the effects of several weeks of endurance training. An apparently trivial soft tissue weakness can lead to an incapacitating injury which may interrupt competition and training for several months. Occasionally the effects of such trauma are permanent.

The provision of a training schedule is only one part of the preparation of an athlete. It is also necessary to ensure that he is free from anatomical and physiological inadequacies which (a) make exercise hazardous, (b) nullify the effects of training, (c) necessitate the use of special types of conditioning regimes, and (d) predispose to injury or other kinds of pathology. In addition it is necessary to provide expert and speedy treatment when problems do arise.

No one individual is likely to possess all the skills necessary to assist the athlete in these matters and ideally the sportsman should have ready access to the following specialists: physician, exercise physiologist, biochemist, nutritionalist, podiatrist, expert in biomechanics, sports psychologist, sports injuries specialist, radiologist and physiotherapist. All need to have current practice relating to the athlete's specialist activity. This latter requirement is absolutely vital if the assistance is to be useful. The requirements of the athlete are so subtle that well meaning advice and treatment from non-specialists can actually be counterproductive. Such assistance is already available to sportsmen in a few countries – those which generally are most successful in international competition. In most other parts of the world the athlete must make do with the advice of his coach, assisted sometimes by the team physician. If this is the case, these individuals will have to assume the roles of all the specialists listed above.

The specific needs of the individual athlete will be influenced by his own characteristics as well as by features of the sport undertaken. For example, it is well known, and not surprising, that lower limb injuries and groin strain are common in soccer players while in rugby players the proportion of upper limb and shoulder problems is higher, and endurance athletes are prone to such conditions as chondromalacia patella (runners knee), shin splints and anaemia. Some of these conditions are preventable; the incidence of others can be lowered or the effects reduced if appropriate precautions are taken.

The first precaution is to ensure that the athlete is basically healthy and fit. The more physiological parts of this type of assessment are considered in detail in Chapter 5, but it is important that the results of all the different testing procedures are integrated since they are all facets of the same picture. Endurance may be influenced by nutrition, cardiorespiratory function and blood biochemistry as well as by training; flexibility and strength are inextricably bound up with the clinical picture of joint and muscle. Thus, if several people are involved in making such assessments it is essential that their efforts be coordinated. Some brief comments on aspects of health and injury prevention appear below.

1. Medical examination

Most types of medical examination will help to ensure that the athlete is free from obvious organic disease and is unlikely to collapse or die during the course of physical activity. This may be reassuring, but a really useful assessment will also have other aims: to identify characteristics which may predispose to injury, or may take the edge off performance, or may lead to situations where these problems could arise at crucial times in the future. Such matters are influenced as much by the various mechanical and physiological stresses generated during different kinds of physical activity as by the clinical characteristics of the athlete. Thus, the interpretation of medical findings in athletes is highly specialised and demands a sound knowledge of biomechanics and the biochemical and physiological adaptions to training. Where this type of help is available it can be of great assistance in the improvement of performance and avoidance of injury.

The actual examination should be as comprehensive as possible since a wide range of conditions have potentially detrimental effects in sport and may not be obvious to the athlete. Poor eyesight has been mistaken for lack of speed in ball-game players slow off the mark, and several metabolic conditions have potentially serious effects upon endurance. The International Committee for the Standardisation of Physical Fitness Tests has produced an outline of a series of clinical and laboratory tests suggested for sportsmen (Kral 1974). These can be adapted to suit the demands of particular activities. If the examination has to be of more limited scope it should address itself to problems common in the athlete's particular sport and to those to which he is known to be predisposed.

The integrity, stability and range of motion of joints is crucial in most sporting activities and all aspects of joint function need to be carefully assessed. Recommendations can then be made regarding treatment, physiotherapy, modifications to the training schedule or the need for supportive strapping. This area is one not well covered in most general examinations. It is also important that muscle function, development and balance be assessed. This aspect of fitness may perhaps be covered by the physiotherapist or coach or through a battery of strength tests. If not it must be included in the medical assessment.

Haematological tests are of considerable importance in sportsmen since anaemia has serious consequences for oxygen transport. Many athletes appear to perform at their best near the lower limit of the normal PCV and haemoglobin ranges but deteriorate badly if their scores

Fig. 2.35 Lung function tests.

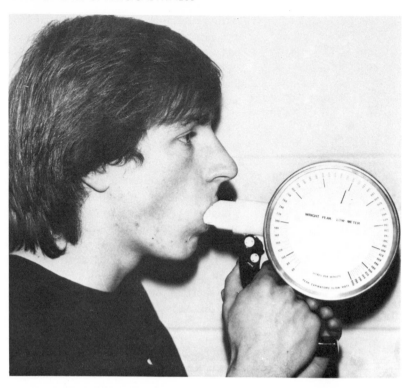

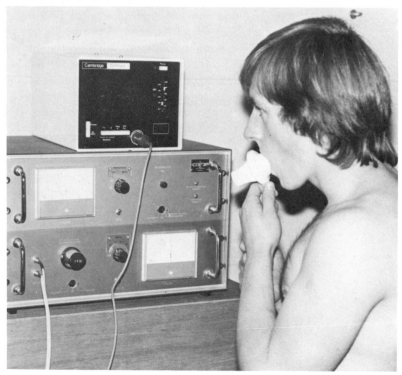

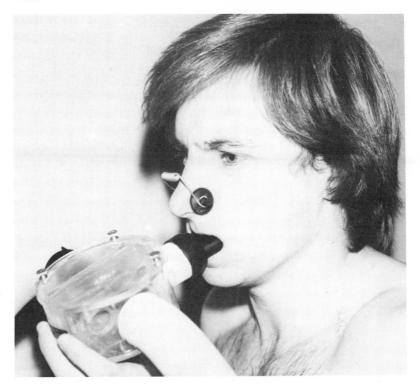

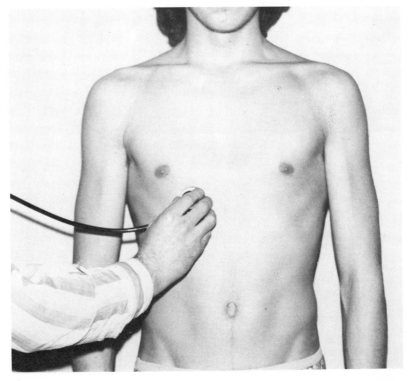

fall a further 3–8 per cent (Watson unpublished). This situation is easily precipitated by an increase in the training load or a slight dietary shortfall. The monitoring of vitamin B_{12}, Folate, TIBC, Transferrin and Ferritin may be useful in susceptible individuals. Levels of serum creatin phosphokinase and lactate dehydrogenase may provide useful information concerning the progress of training, but interpretation is difficult as the levels in many sportsmen are far above the normal range. Levels of haemoglobin and protein in urine are also often abnormal. In a few athletes the work of breathing is excessive at high ventilation rates and respiratory function tests can be useful. Unless a specialised nutritionalist is available the physician may also be requested to advise in this area.

2 Fitness

Adequate fitness is important in minimising the risk of sports injury. The topic has been considered elsewhere but the need for strength,

Fig. 2.36 Medical aspects of fitness: ECG, testing urine for blood and protein, examination of the lower limb, application of strapping for support of the knee.

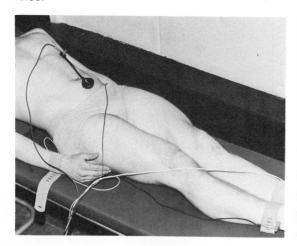
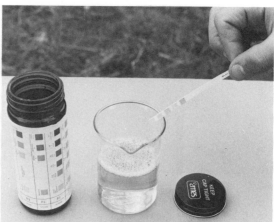
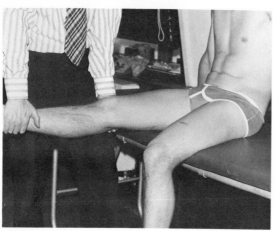
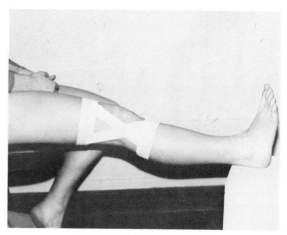

muscle balance and flexibility is stressed. Poor endurance leads to early fatigue which increases the risk of injury.

3. Nutrition (see p. 58)

4. Posture – body and foot mechanics
Defects cause abnormal stresses on particular muscles and ligaments and increase the risk of injury (see p. 57 and the section on Footwear below).

5. Supportive strapping
Weak and recently injured joints should always be supported, even during training. Supportive strapping is not widely used in many European countries but can considerably reduce the risk of injury. To be effective it must support the joint along the line of weakness while allowing unhindered movement in all other directions. Elastic knee and ankle bandages provide only psychological support.

6. Kit and equipment
The kit and equipment should be designed for the sport in question; it should also be clean, well fitting and in good condition. The equipment should be checked for any defects that may cause accidents.

7. Playing areas
Where applicable these should be dry, even and well lit. Wet indoor surfaces are particularly dangerous. The periphery of the playing area should be free of hazardous objects. Avoid hard surfaces during training.

8. Footwear
Footwear provides traction, protection and support. Training shoes should be light, comfortable and flexible while providing adequate heel support and having good shock absorbing characteristics in the sole and heel. The latter requirement will vary with the individual's body weight and the type of surface used for training. Adequate traction in the sole is also important. In some cases raising the heel or increasing the arch support helps to avoid certain 'over-use' injuries.

9. Warm-up
This is essential (*see p. 79*).

10. Safety precautions
These are mainly common sense, but are frequently ignored. Protective equipment appropriate to particular activities should always be used. All appropriate safety precautions should be vigorously observed. If necessary steps should be taken against reckless players and incompetent referees or other officials. Athletes should decline to take part in activities if conditions are not considered safe.

11. First aid

Prompt and appropriate first aid minimises the seriousness of injuries and considerably reduces recovery time. Someone experienced in the first aid management of sports injuries should always be available and be provided with appropriate equipment. This should include: Scoop stretcher, cervical collar, air splints, ice packs, compression bandages, sterile dressings, a selection of other bandages, and blankets.

12. Medical treatment

When an injury occurs the athlete needs speedy access to expert medical help. The service provided by many hospital casualty departments is

Fig. 2.37 *Top*: common sites of injury on the leg and muscle atrophy following lower leg injury. *Bottom*: satisfactory and poor footwear, blood analysis.

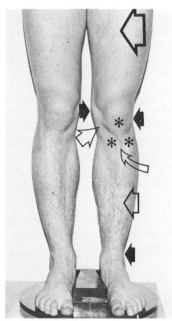
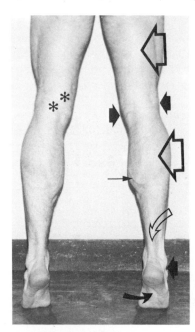
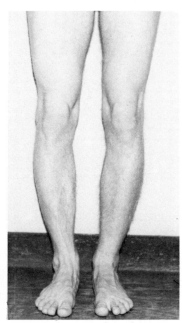

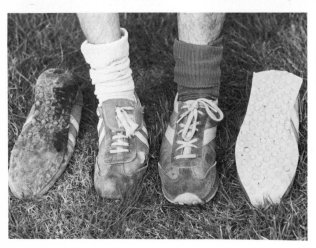

ESR	M 1 — 5 F 4 — 7	*10*			
32 — 36	MCHC	*34.0* g/dl		Neut	*70*
				Stabs	
27 — 33	MCH	*27.8* pg		Lymphs	*24*
				Monos	
76 — 96	MCV	*092* fl		Eos	*6*
M. 40 — .54 F. 36 — .47	PCV	*0.382* I/I		Metamyelo	
				Baso	
M. 14 — 18 F. 12 — 16	Hb	*13.0* g/dl		Retics	
M. 4.5 — 6.5 F. 4.0 — 5.5	RBC	*4.66* x10¹²			
WBC	WBC	*13.4* x10⁹		Monospot	
150 — 400	PLTS (+WBC)	*23.1* x10⁹		*10*	

often inadequate and a few are unsympathetic to the injured athlete. Bone and joint injuries should always be seen by an orthopaedic surgeon. The situation is often worse when chronic injuries occur. In any particular district there may be no-one with adequate experience of diagnosing and treating such conditions.

13. Rehabilitation

After injury rehabilitation is vital if recovery is to be complete and re-injury avoided. Weakened muscles and ligaments must be strengthened and joint mobility restored. This must be accomplished gradually and demands the cooperation of athlete, physiotherapist and coach.

Fig. 2.38 a) Foul play, a frequent source of injury. b) Sustaining a contusion. c) First aid equipment. d) Mild scoliosis in a hand-ball player.

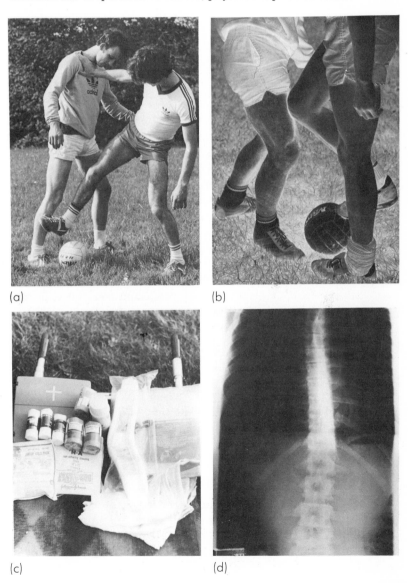

(a)

(b)

(c)

(d)

3 FEATURES OF TRAINING, WARM-UP, MOTOR UNIT TYPES

TRAINING

ADAPTION

If you regularly take your Mini up the motorway at top speed one of two things will eventually happen. The car will either expire in a noisy disintegration of half-shafts, big-ends and cylinder-head gasket; or its top speed will gradually decline as the engine loses its tune and begins to wear. If you run regularly at top speed yourself the result is likely to be different. A catastrophic disintegration is still possible but provided you remain intact your top speed will slowly increase. This improvement is due to the effects of training.

The human body differs from a mechanical engine in that it can sometimes adapt to certain conditions. In this respect it is like a thermostatically controlled central heating system which responds to cold weather by producing more heat; in other ways the body is different and much more complex. An appreciation of the process of adaption is essential to an understanding of the effects of training.

The body responds only to certain types of stimuli. Weight-lifting leads to the development of larger muscles, and running produces a greater stroke volume of the heart. But high-jumping does not lead to an increase in leg length or interval training to a higher maximum heart rate, although both these changes would be advantageous. They do not occur because the body has no biological mechanism capable of bringing them about. Some of the biochemical and physiological adaptions that occur during training were considered in Chapter 2.

OVERLOAD

A training effect usually occurs when a part of the body is worked harder than normal. The situation is often referred to as 'overload'. Biological changes then occur and endurance fitness or strength is increased. In general terms the size of the training effect depends upon the degree of overload. If the muscles are used to raise weights only slightly heavier than those normally lifted, the training effect is small. If heavier weights are used, strength gains are more rapid.

There is a definite intensity of effort below which no training effect occurs. This varies from person to person depending mainly upon the individual's initial capacity, as illustrated in Fig. 3.1.

Fig. 3.1 The overload principle. The bottom portion of the diagram indicates that 100 kg could be lifted prior to training. Using 75 per cent of this as a training load (75 kg) produces considerable overload and a large increase in strength results (right-hand diagram). 50 kg produces less overload and a lower increase in strength (centre). Training with 25 kg produces no overload and no gains in strength occur.

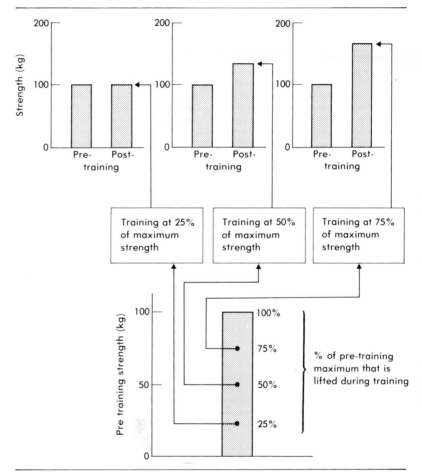

If the person can lift 100 kg with a particular muscle group, a moderate training effect is produced if he trains with 50 per cent of this weight. If he trains with 75 kg the gains in strength are larger. There is no significant training effect when very small weights are lifted.

As the training proceeds the individual becomes stronger and 75 kg is no longer 75 per cent of his maximum lift. He will now need to train with a heavier weight if the strength gains are to continue at the same rate as before. This is illustrated in Fig. 3.2.

The situation with other aspects of fitness is similar. As the individual increases his fitness the absolute intensity of the exercise must be increased correspondingly in order to maintain the overload.

Fig. 3.2 The effects of training with different percentages of the maximum lift. The subject's initial strength is 100 kg. Training with 25 kg produces no overload and strength does not increase however long the subject trains (a). If the subject begins his training by lifting 75 kg, strength is gained more rapidly than with 50 kg (b). If he continues to train with 75 kg the gains become slower (c) and eventually stop (d). For maximum increases the training load should be raised to keep pace with the strength gains (e).

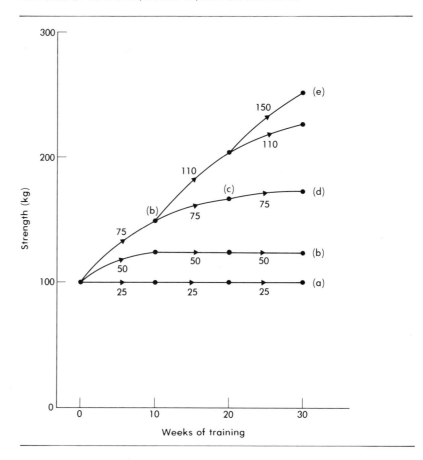

SPECIFICITY

The effects of training are confined to those systems, or parts of systems, actually subject to overload. Thus, running does little or nothing to improve strength; neither does weight-lifting normally increase flexibility. Furthermore, strength training will affect only the muscles actually involved in the exercise and the gains may be confined to the movements that occur during training. After isometric exercise increases in strength may be confined to the joint angles used during contraction and there may be little or no increase in the capacity for isotonic work. Increases in anaerobic endurance, due to changes in the concentration of high-energy phosphate compounds and associated enzymes, are also confined to the muscles actually trained. Likewise, gains in flexibility occur only in the joints that are actually exercised. Cardiovascular fitness is slightly more general in that the heart and major blood vessels service all the tissues; but even here there is a great deal of specificity because training produces biochemical changes in the muscles that are active, and capillary density is also increased (Pettengale and Holloszy 1967; Gollnick and King 1969; Benzi *et al*. 1975). All types of aerobic training lead to similar changes in blood volume and cardiac function, but the local changes are confined to the trained muscles and exercise involving running will not lead to an optimum improvement in the oxygen uptake during swimming where a different set of muscles is involved (see p. 114).

As a general principle it is an advantage if the athlete can train in a manner that simulates his competitive activity as closely as possible. Overload can be obtained by making the activity a little more difficult.

It may be necessary to remind the sportsman that the specificity of training is determined by the biochemistry of his own cells, not by his coach or the editor of his favourite athletics magazine. An exercise may appear to be specific to a particular manoeuvre, but that is no guarantee that it is of any value as a method of training. The only really satisfactory way of evaluating a new conditioning procedure is by means of a carefully controlled experimental study which includes an examination of the biochemical changes. A knowledge of some of the principles of training physiology will help the athlete to avoid advice that is unsound, even though it may be well-intentioned.

CROSS-TRANSFER

Despite the remarks of the previous section some cross-transfer effects of training do occur. This is because the different organs and tissues of the body are not entirely separate and the effects of a particular type of training will not be exclusively confined to one part of the body. Also, it is difficult to overload one area of the body without putting some extra stress on other parts. Endurance running is not a good method of developing the strength of the legs. However, an individual who undertakes this exercise regularly may develop greater leg strength than a person who takes no exercise at all.

The term **cross-transfer** is commonly applied to the strength gains occurring in one limb when the opposite one is trained. This phenomenon was first described in 1894 (Scripture *et al*. 1894). In a fairly typical study it was found that the untrained arm increased in strength by 8.9 per cent following a programme of training that produced a 12.6 per cent increase in the trained arm (Shaver 1975). The effect is usually attributed to motor impulses arriving at the muscles of the inactive as well as the exercising limb. These may cause isometric contractions in the muscles of the limb which is not being trained (Rasch and Morehouse 1957; Hellebrandt 1958; Wellock 1958). The cross-transfer effects of training are usually much less significant than the primary result. For optimum gains in fitness it is essential that training programmes are tailored to the aspects of fitness which need to be developed.

REVERSAL

The effects of training are not permanent and when physical activity is discontinued fitness drops towards the pre-training level. The regression is usually less rapid than the initial increase and a given level of fitness can often be retained with a much lower level of training than was needed for its development. Differences in the level of activity between individuals make it difficult to quantify the rate of reversal once training has stopped. After short training programmes strength seems to be lost at a rate of 0.3–1 per cent of the gains each week (Müller and Hettinger 1954; McMorris and Elkins 1954); that is, if the individual resumes his normal pre-training activity. If the limb is totally immobilised the losses may be up to 5 per cent *per day* (Müller 1970). This vast difference illustrates the importance of the level of post-training activity on the retention of strength. Berger (1965) has shown that one set of maximum contractions per week is enough to maintain strength and may even lead to further gains. With a normal level of activity losses are often small in the first week. After this there is a more rapid decline for 4–6 weeks, then the losses become more gradual (Shaver 1975).

Endurance fitness also declines when appropriate training is stopped. The decline is gradual and the higher the level that is achieved through training the longer the effects continue. Smith and Stransky (1976) found that an 8 per cent gain, achieved over 7 weeks, disappeared 7 weeks after training was stopped. In another study 10–14 per cent gains in $\dot{V}_{O_2max}$ were reversed after 7 weeks (Penderson and Jorgensen 1978). A group of champion oarsmen retained 82 per cent of their maximum oxygen intake 18 months after training had stopped (Hagermann *et al.* 1975). This suggests that they had probably retained about half the gains achieved through endurance training.

But even very high levels of fitness eventually decline. A group of champion middle-distance athletes, whose maximum oxygen uptake was once 41 per cent above average, were only 14 per cent above average 25 years later. Most of these men were still doing some running. The $\dot{V}_{O_2max}$ of two who had become sedentary was below the average for their age group (Robinson *et al.* 1976). The study again demonstrates the influence of post-training activity on the rate of decline of fitness.

Some features of the reversal of training are summarised in Fig. 3.3. The rate of decline is normally lower than the rate of increase but is influenced by the post-training activity level. The decline can often be halted by quite small amounts of further training. With a normal level of activity a fit individual (subject A) will maintain some of his gains for many weeks or months. When the gains due to training are small (subject B), they are likely to disappear in a short time. The aspects of fitness that are acquired slowly are generally retained for the longest period. Structural changes in muscle will persist for many months, perhaps even years, while functional changes and increases in blood volume are reversed more quickly. Thus, it appears that the structural aspects of endurance fitness can be built up over a number of years, although the functional part will still be influenced by the state of training at a given time. It is known that gains of 15–20 per cent can be brought about relatively quickly while larger increases take much

Fig. 3.3 The acquisition and reversal of fitness. Subject A trains for 25 weeks. This results in a large increase in fitness. The rate of reversal of these gains depends upon his subsequent level of activity. Quite small amounts of further training may lead to the gains being retained. Subject B acquires small fitness gains over a five-week period. These are soon reversed when the training is stopped.

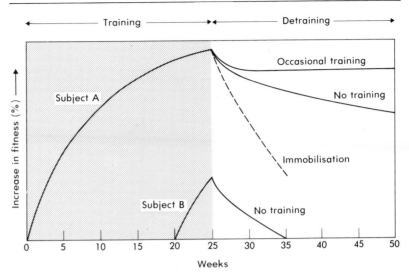

longer to occur (Astrand and Rodahl 1970; Kilbom 1971). Structural changes in muscle, due to strength training, also persist for a considerable time. Very high levels of strength must be acquired over a number of years and are then well retained.

INTERFERENCE

Hickson (1980) has recently investigated the effects of training for strength and aerobic endurance simultaneously. Increases in aerobic capacity occurred at the same rate as in subjects who undertook this kind of training alone, but gains in strength were significantly less than in a group undertaking only weight training. Hickson concludes that endurance training 'interferes' with strength training.

What can be achieved through training
The limits of achievement through training are set by the opportunities available and the genetic endowment of the individual. The effects of training have been most widely studied in relation to aerobic capacity. The maximum possible improvement for a sedentary individual appears to be between 25 and 35 per cent, considerably less for someone who is already semi-trained (Astrand and Rodahl 1970; Shephard 1969). The range of maximum oxygen uptake scores found in the general population is shown in Fig. 3.4. Scores for champion endurance athletes are also given. The effect of a 35 per cent improvement on various values is indicated. It is clear than an average sedentary individual cannot expect to raise his maximum oxygen uptake to the level of a champion endurance athlete, however hard he trains. Only if he has a value of about 60 ml kg^{-1}. min^{-1} while sedentary has he much hope of becoming a champion cross-country skier.

75

Fig. 3.4 Changes in maximum oxygen uptake with training. The normal range for males is shown at the bottom of the diagram. Gains are limited to 20–30 per cent of the initial value. Even with maximum training it is not possible for most individuals to achieve the values of champion athletes.

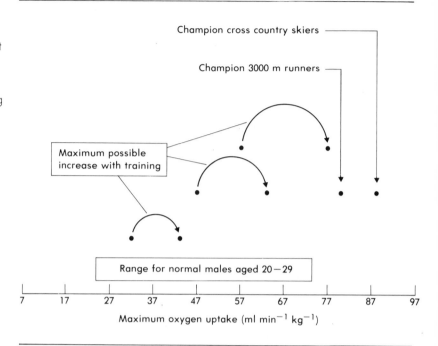

The limitations on other types of training have been less extensively studied but it is clear that strength can be improved to a much greater degree than aerobic capacity. Gains of several hundred per cent are common and champion weight-lifters probably achieve even more.

Comparisons of pairs of identical twins are a useful way of assessing the influence of genetic factors on aspects of fitness and physical performance. Such studies indicate that lung size and respiratory function during exercise are influenced by genetic factors (Man and Zamel 1975). It has also been shown that pairs of identical twins have sporting interests and activity patterns that are much closer than those of non-identical twins. In a study on adolescent twins it was shown that 93 per cent of the variations in maximum oxygen uptake were attributable to genetic factors (Klissouras 1971). Other studies have shown a strong genetic element in hand-grip, back strength, dynamic balance, time for a 1 km run and anaerobic capacity (Venerando and Milani-Comaretti 1970; Williams and Hearfield 1973; Klissouras 1973; Montoye *et al.* 1975).

Performance is improved by training but it appears that the upper limit of most performance variables is set by genetic factors. This has led Astrand to the conclusion: 'I am convinced that anyone interested in winning Olympic gold medals must select his or her parents very carefully' (Astrand 1967). Some of the factors favourable to four specific types of athletic event are illustrated in Fig. 3.5.

Fig. 3.5 Factors favourable to performance in four different athletic events: long-distance running, high jump, sprinting, shot-put.

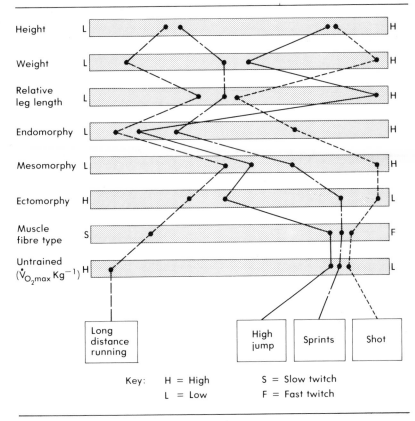

Key: H = High   S = Slow twitch
        L = Low   F = Fast twitch

FACTORS WHICH AFFECT TRAINING

The rate of improvement in fitness may be influenced by several factors, including: the initial level of fitness; the age, sex and nutritional status of the individual; the mode, frequency, intensity and duration of training; the genetic endowment of the individual.

Initial level of fitness

The initial level of fitness has an important influence on the gains likely to be obtained through training. Figure 3.7 shows pre- and post-training scores of a group of 16 schoolboys who undertook the same programme of endurance training. The programme consisted of 200 m interval running and was carefully supervised so that each individual undertook exactly the same amount of exercise. The subjects with the lowest pre-training scores increased their physical working capacity while those who were fittest at the start of the study showed no improvement. This is because the training did not produce an overload in the fitter subjects who had undertaken other types of endurance training previously. Even when overload does occur, increases are usually slower in subjects who have already undertaken some training.

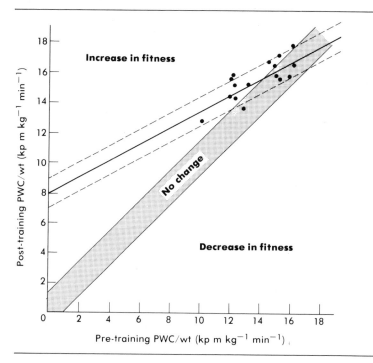

Fig. 3.6 The effects of initial level of fitness on the results of a training programme. Sixteen subjects undertook interval training for five weeks. Their post-training physical working capacities are plotted on the vertical axis against the initial value on the horizontal axis. All individuals with an initial score of 12 units or less increased their physical working capacities as a result of training. The majority of those with a pre-training score of 14 units or above failed to improve. (From Watson and O'Donovan 1977b.)

The influence of initial level of fitness on the rate of increase often causes difficulties in interpreting the results of training programmes. If you devise a new type of endurance programme and test it on discharged hospital patients you will probably get spectacular results. Many of the claims for 'instant fitness' programmes are based on just this type of study. They usually give disappointing results when used with sportsmen who are already in good condition.

Intensity, duration, frequency
These are considered in more detail in connection with specific types of programme but some general points are noted here.

The intensity of training must be sufficient to produce overload otherwise no gains in fitness occur. When overload has been reached the training effect appears to depend upon a combination of intensity and duration, provided the latter is neither very short nor very long. Many older studies appeared to overestimate the contribution of intensity. Some recent investigations suggest that the two factors may play a more equal part.

The frequency of training also seems to have a general effect. Small gains in most components of fitness have been noted following one training session per week. Two or three sessions per week normally produce much more significant increases, and are usually recommended at the start of a training programme. Raising the number to four or five may lead to a further improvement, but this does not always occur.

Where there are three or four training sessions per week it is usually recommended that they take place on alternate days. Many authors suggest that training on consecutive days is less effective. Only one systematic investigation of this proposition is known. Moffatt *et al.* (1977) compared the effects of endurance training on three consecutive days with the same training carried out on Monday, Wednesday and Friday. They found no difference in the gains in maximum oxygen uptake and conclude that the *placement* of tri-weekly training sessions is unimportant.

Age

The effects of a programme of training may be influenced by the subject's age and developmental status. A number of studies have failed to detect any increase in the maximum oxygen uptake per kilogram of body weight of young schoolboys following endurance training (Sprynarova 1966; Ekblom 1969; Cumming *et al.* 1969; Daniels and Oldbridge 1971; Hamilton and Andrews 1976; Daniels *et al.* 1978a). This has not been a completely universal finding (see Eriksson 1969 and Shephard 1977) but it is clear that up to the end of puberty the effects of training are much less marked. The physical capabilities of children appear to be determined primarily by considerations of size, and growth is a more important influence than training. In a recent study by Weber *et al.* (1976) it was found that a group of 16-year-olds responded to training but 13-year-olds, who were growing rapidly, did not. A group of 10-year-olds responded to a small extent. There is little evidence to support the idea that training has a particularly marked and long-term effect in the young. In fact, the opposite is nearer the truth.

In children and adolescents both strength and aerobic capacity are strongly influenced by size (Watson and O'Donovan 1977a; Davies *et al.* 1972). As age increases this relationship gradually declines and the effects of training become more significant. It was once thought that training had a reduced effect as the subject aged. More recent studies show that this is not the case, and that endurance training produces a similar percentage increase in aerobic capacity in individuals aged 50–80 as in younger subjects (De Vries 1970; Adams and De Vries 1973; Suominen *et al.* 1977).

WARM-UP

A period of preparatory activity undertaken before the start of a race or match is known as a **warm-up**. A warm-up of an appropriate nature normally enhances physical performance by increasing: (1) joint mobility and flexibility; (2) the power output available from muscles; (3) coordination; and (4) the energy available from aerobic metabolism at the start of activity so that less energy is derived from the production of lactic acid. The susceptibility to injury is also reduced. These effects are derived from different types of warm-up and individuals sometimes show a variable response. These points are considered below.

FLEXIBILITY

A short period of light stretching exercise is capable of increasing flexibility, presumably by its effect upon the length and suppleness of muscle and other tissues. This type of warm-up should be undertaken by everyone about to engage in physical activity.

POWER OUTPUT

The power output of a muscle is increased when its temperature is raised (Binkhorst *et al.* 1977). This is illustrated in Fig. 2.32, p. 54. The effect probably occurs for three reasons: (1) muscle viscosity is reduced; (2) the speed of conduction of impulses by nerves is increased (Zuntz *et al.* 1906); and (3) the rate of chemical reactions is increased. It is necessary to raise muscle temperature by about 2 degC before these effects become significant. A fairly strenuous warm-up lasting several minutes is therefore required in order to optimise power output.

COORDINATION

Coordination improves after a few minutes of practice. When an activity involves fine motor skills these should be rehearsed during the period of warm-up.

AEROBIC METABOLISM

An adequate warm-up increases the rate of aerobic metabolism at the start of exercise. This has the effect of decreasing the contribution of anaerobic processes, thereby minimising the accumulation of lactic acid. This is illustrated in Fig. 3.7 which shows the effect of a warm-up, consisting of 15 minutes of strenuous running, on a well-trained athlete.

The warm-up produced five changes: (1) muscle temperature was increased; (2) oxygen intake rose more rapidly at the start of exercise and (3) reached a higher maximum value; (4) as a consequence of (2) and (3) less energy was obtained from anaerobic sources so that the concentration of blood lactate was lower; and (5), as Fig. 3.7. also shows, the heart rate rose more rapidly after warm-up. The physiological changes that accompany this kind of warm-up are many and complex. Hormones which are secreted into the bloodstream enhance cardiac function and cause blood to be diverted to the working muscles. Activity in the autonomic nervous system has a similar effect. This results in a greater blood flow to skeletal muscle and a cardiovascular system that is more responsive to sudden demands. The increase in muscle temperature is also important: it reduces the affinity of haemoglobin for oxygen and permits more of this gas to be released from a given volume of blood; it also enhances the rate of aerobic reactions inside muscle cells, and thus has a similar effect on oxygen uptake. This results in more

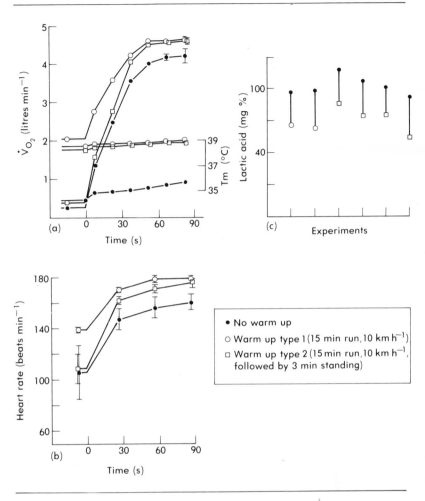

Fig. 3.7 The effects of warm-up on oxygen uptake, blood lactate concentration and heart-rate during subsequent exercise. Data for one subject from Martin *et al.* (1975), by kind permission of the authors.

oxygen being extracted from a given volume of inhaled air so that the cost-effectiveness of breathing is improved (Ingjer and Strømme 1979). There also seem to be psychological effects that occur even if the warm-up is physiologically ineffective (Malarecki 1954).

In order to produce these changes the warm-up must consist of 15–30 minutes of heavy activity. This must be strenuous enough to produce sweating. Passive warm-up, by means of hot baths or showers, has little, if any, effect (Ingjer and Stromme 1979). It seems that only fit individuals are able to benefit. Apparently the poorly conditioned lack the cardiovascular and cellular adaption necessary for an intensive warm-up to be effective (Knowlton and Miles 1978). This is probably an academic point because only well-trained individuals will be capable of completing such a warm-up without becoming exhausted. It is one of the reasons why a reasonable level of all-round fitness is necessary for anyone seeking a high level of physical performance.

THE TRANSITION FROM EXERCISE TO RECOVERY

Recovery from heavy physical activity is facilitated if the transition is made gradually. This phase of exercise is variously known as 'warm-down', 'cool-down' or 'recovery'. Lactic acid is metabolised more rapidly during moderate activity than at rest. Also, cardiac function is better maintained. During exercise much of the venous return to the heart is achieved by the action of contracting skeletal muscle on limb veins. If physical activity is halted suddenly a great deal of blood remains in the limbs and cardiac function is seriously impaired.

MOTOR UNIT TYPES – MUSCLE FIBRE TYPES

Skeletal muscle consists of a number of different types of muscle fibre. These have distinct mechanical and chemical properties including the tension that can be developed during a maximum contraction, the time taken for contraction, the resistance to fatigue, and the concentration of different enzymes and other biologically active chemicals. In addition, different types of fibre are innervated by distinct varieties of motor neurone which have a crucial role in determining how the muscle fibre behaves. Thus, skeletal muscle consists of a number of different types of motor unit (see Chapter 2 for a description of motor unit). The distribution of motor unit types varies from individual to individual and has an important influence upon physical performance.

This is a confusing area because there are several ways of classifying muscle fibres. They can be grouped in terms of mechanical properties, such as twitch-speed, or by their biochemical and histological characteristics. There is a good deal of overlap between the systems because mechanical properties are, to a large extent, determined by the structure and biochemistry of the fibre. The best-known system classifies fibres as either 'red – slow twitch fibres with high endurance' or 'white – fast twitch fibres with low endurance'. It is actually possible to distinguish up to eight different types of fibre. Of these, three are of particular importance. These can be designated either in terms of their mechanical properties or their biochemical profile. A number designation is also frequently used. Classifications that are essentially similar are listed in Table 3.1, and the principal properties of the three types of fibre are given in Table 3.2.

TYPE I FIBRES (S OR SO)

These are the classical 'red' muscle fibres. They contract relatively slowly, have low maximum tension and high endurance. They are rich in mitochrondria, oxidative enzymes and capillary supply and have a low concentration of myofibrillar ATP-ase and glycolytic enzymes (Burke and Edgerton 1975). They tend to contain a type of lactate dehydrogenase adapted for the conversion of lactic acid into pyruvic acid

Table 3.1 Equivalent systems of classifying muscle fibres

Motor unit designation	Slow twitch	Fast twitch, fatigue resistant (FR)	Fast twitch, fatiguable (FF)
Biochemical designation	Slow twitch, oxidative (SO)	Fast twitch, oxidative, glycolytic (FOG)	Fast twitch, glycolytic (FG)
Number designation	I	IIa	IIb
Other designation	Slow twitch, red	Fast twitch, intermediate	Fast twitch, white

By courtesy of J. T. Fitzgerald.

Table 3.2

	IIb	IIa	I
Motor neurone properties			
Speed of conduction (m s^{-1})	85–114	84–113	75–99
Mechanical properties			
Twitch contraction time (m s^{-1})	20–47	30–55	58–110
Maximum tension (g)	30–130	4.5–55	1.2–12.6
Resistance to fatigue	Low	High	Very high
Mean fibre area (μ^2)	5,290	2,890	1,730
Biochemical properties			
Myofibrillar ATP-ase	High	High	Low
AC–ATP-ase	High	Intermediate	Low
Glycolytic enzymes	High	High	Low
Oxidative enzymes	Low	Intermediate	High
Myoglobin content	Low	High	High
Other features			
Capillary supply	Poor	Abundant	Abundant
Colour	White	Reddish	Reddish

(Peter *et al.* 1971); thus they specialise in removing the lactic acid produced by other types of fibre (see p. 37). They are used during activities involving low muscle tension (Milner-Brown *et al.* 1973).

TYPE IIB FIBRES (FF OR FG)

These are the classical 'white' fibres and have properties that are practically the reverse of type I. They are used for 'strength' and 'explosive' type activities and are not activated during low-tension work (Warmolts and Engel 1973).

TYPE IIA FIBRES (FR OR FOG)

These are intermediate type fibres. They have mechanical properties similar to type IIb but have a higher concentration of oxidative enzymes and a better blood supply. Consequently, they are considerably more resistant to fatigue. Type IIa fibres are red in colour and fast-twitch in mechanical properties. The properties of a muscle fibre seem to be principally determined by the type of motor neurone innervating it (Guth 1968; Salmons and Vrbova 1969; Pette *et al.* 1973). Extraneous factors, such as training, can influence function only within the limits set by the basic fibre type. Not enough work has been done in this area to be categorical, but it seems that the effects of certain sorts of training may be restricted to particular fibre types. Strength training seems to cause hypertrophy of fast-twitch fibres (principally type IIb) with much less effect on slow-twitch fibres (type I) and the oxidative capacity of muscle (Gollnick et al. 1972; MacDougall et al. 1980). The cross-sectional area of fast-twitch fibres is increased but not the total number of fibres. Endurance training seems to have a different effect. Following six months of such a programme Gollnich et al. (1973) found a 24 per cent enlargement of the slow-twitch fibres with no significant change in the area of the fast-twitch type. It is well documented that endurance training increases the concentration of oxidative enzymes (see Ch. 2). It seems likely that an individual's capacity for oxygen uptake (his maximum oxygen uptake) is considerably influenced by the percentage of slow-twitch fibres (type I) (Bergh et al. 1978).

Type IIa fibres (FOG) differ from the FG variety (type IIb) mainly in terms of enzyme concentrations. There is some evidence that endurance training can lead to a conversion of type FG fibres to FOG (Edgerton et al. 1969; Barnard et al. 1970). This does not amount to a change in mechanical properties since both are of the fast-twitch type. There seems to be no evidence to suggest that fast-twitch fibres can be converted to the slow-twitch type or vice-versa.

It has been demonstrated that strength and the speed of muscle contraction are related to the percentage of fast-twitch fibres (Thorstensson et al. 1976). As might be expected, the relationship between strength and percentage of fast-twitch fibres is particularly marked when the speed of contraction is high (Coyle et al. 1979). Also, Bosco and Komi (1979) have shown that power output is related to muscle fibre composition.

4 TRAINING METHODS

STRENGTH

There are a number of different ways of training for strength. The features of some of the more common methods are summarised in Table 4.1.

The last two methods given in the table are relatively straightforward and do not involve the purchase of expensive items of equipment. The

Table 4.1 Features of different types of strength training

Type	Features	Other names commonly used
Isometric	Muscle develops tension against the resistance of an immovable object; no movement occurs	Static resistance
Weight-lifting*	A weight is lifted and tension is developed as the muscle shortens	Isotonic, concentric, constant resistance
Eccentric weight training	A weight is slowly lowered and tension is developed as the muscle lengthens	Negative work training
Variable resistance weight training	The resistance of the weight is applied to the limb via a cam; this is designed to allow the muscle to develop maximum tension throughout its range of movement	Nautilus training
Accommodating resistance training	The resistance to motion is varied mechanically in response to the speed of movement	Isokinetic, constant speed training
Exercise with spring devices	Resistance is supplied by springs and increases as these are extended or compressed	
Dynamic exercises	Muscles are usually exercised using body weight as a resistance	

* If the weight is lowered slowly, eccentric muscular contraction also occurs.

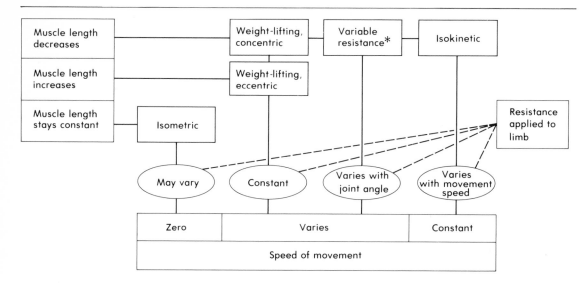

*In this type of training the tension developed by the muscle is approximately constant throughout the range of movement

Fig. 4.1 Characteristics of the muscular contraction occurring during various types of strength training. Speed of movement, nature of the resistance to movement and changes in muscle length are shown for the five principal types of strength training.

other four each employ a particular type of muscular contraction. Some of the characteristics of these are illustrated in Fig. 4.1.

Weight-lifting and isometric exercises are the traditional methods of increasing strength. Other types of training have been introduced more recently in an attempt to take account of certain physiological principles discussed in Chapter 2.

WEIGHT-LIFTING

This can be undertaken either with a set of weights or by using a weight-training machine. In both cases the subject normally lifts a weight, then lowers it. Thus one lift usually consists of a concentric contraction followed by an eccentric one. The weight-training machine replicates many of the exercises possible with a set of weights and also provides additional exercises. It is an expensive item of equipment but has advantages in terms of speed and safety. Although the two methods of weight-training are essentially similar, there are some important differences. The maximum range of movement may vary; there may be slight differences in the muscle groups used for a particular exercise; a weight-training machine tends to confine lifts to a smaller number of muscles. On many machines arm exercises are executed by pushing on a bar, so that there is little involvement of the hand-grip muscles. Weight-training has its own distinctive terminology, and some of the more commonly used terms are explained in Table 4.2.

Most modern weight-training programmes are based on a model put forward by De Lorme and Watkins (1948, 1951). This consisted of three sets of exercises, each set containing 10 repetitions. The training

Table 4.2 Some terms used in weight training

Term	Meaning	Example
Lift	A particular way of moving a weight	The arm curl. In this lift the weight is moved by flexion at the elbows
Repetition	One execution of a lift or exercise against a resistance	Lifting a weight and lowering it once
Number of repetitions	The number of repetitions performed consecutively	
Set	A group of repetitions followed by a rest or change of activity	Six arm curls followed by a rest would constitute one set. In theory there is no limit to the number of repetitions in a set. In practice a number between 1 and 20 is usually used
Repetition maximum (R.M.)	The maximum weight that can be lifted a specified number of times with a particular type of lift	If subject X can manage 5 repetitions with a 100 lb weight, his 5 R.M. is 100 lb. If Y can perform 10 repetitions with a 100 lb weight, his 10 R.M. is 100 lb.
Training load	The weight or resistance employed Often specified in terms of the R.M.	50% of 10 R.M. This is half the weight that the individual can lift 10 times
Training frequency	The number of training sessions per week	
Training programme	A prescription specifying some, or all, of the parameters above.	

load was based on the subject's 10 repetition maximum (10 R.M.). This is the weight that the subject can just lift 10 times, and was determined before the training started. The first set of exercises consisted of 10 repetitions of a load that was 50 per cent of the 10 R.M. This was followed by a second set of 10 repetitions at 75 per cent of the 10 R.M. The final set consisted of 10 repetitions at 100% of the 10 R.M. The programme is summarised below.

De Lorme and Watkins progression for an individual with a 10 repetition maximum of 100 lb.

Set 1   10 repetitions with 50% of 10 R.M.   (50 lb)
Set 2   10 repetitions with 75% of 10 R.M.   (75 lb)
Set 3   10 repetitions with 100% of 10 R.M.   (100 lb)

The repetitions in a particular set were undertaken consecutively with a short rest between sets. A training frequency of four or five times per week was recommended.

As the training proceeded the individual became stronger and the 10 RM was increased. When more than 10 repetitions of a particular lift could be completed the weight was increased to the new 10 R.M. load (see Fig. 3.3).

There have been several more recent investigations into strength-training procedures. These have generally examined the effect of variations in the load and number of repetitions. The greater the load, the lower the number of repetitions possible. If an individual can lift a given weight 10 times he can usually manage a slightly heavier one 8 or 9 times. The maximum weight increases as the number of repetitions is reduced. The maximum weight for a given number of repetitions is known as the 'repetition maximum', i.e. 6 R.M. is the maximum load that can just be lifted 6 times.

Work by Berger (1962a, 1963) suggests that, on average, maximum gains are likely with three sets of lifts each at about 6 RM. Other studies suggest that optimum results occur with R.M.s between 3 and 9 (Berger 1962b; Withers 1970).

The effect of training frequency on the rate of strength gain has not been extensively studied. The majority of contemporary writers recommend a frequency of three or four times per week with rest days between. Some athletes train six days a week but confine work on particular parts of the body to alternate days.

ECCENTRIC WEIGHT TRAINING

Eccentric contraction occurs when a muscle develops force in order to resist being lengthened. It is a feature of any activity in which a heavy object is slowly lowered to the ground. Eccentric contraction of muscle then resists the force exerted on the object by gravity. This occurs during weight training if the load is slowly lowered back to its starting position.

Eccentric contraction is an effective means of producing increases in muscular strength. The gains seem to be identical to those obtained with the same amount of concentric work (Seleger *et al*. 1968; Johnson 1972; Johnson *et al*. 1976). To make the most of a weight-training session the weights should be slowly lowered back to the starting position. Providing this is done *slowly*, eccentric work ought to contribute as much to the development of strength as the concentric contractions that occurred when the weights were raised.

Heavier weights can be used for eccentric training than are possible with concentric work. If 100 lb is the maximum concentric lift, a weight of 120 lb can normally be controlled during lowering. Johnson *et al*. (1976) found that six eccentric contractions at 120 per cent of the concentric 1 R.M. produced the same training effect as 10 concentric lifts at 80 per cent of the 1 R.M.. If more than 120 per cent of the concentric 1 R.M. is used, the individual has difficulty controlling the weight, which falls rapidly. The gains in strength are then minimal.

Eccentric training appears to have two possible advantages. Johnson *et al*. (1976) report that their subjects found eccentric training easier than an equivalent amount of concentric training. Second, it can sometimes be used where concentric work is impossible. During circuit training some individuals cannot perform even one push-up or chin. If they begin training by lowering themselves the eccentric work leads to strength gains so that they can eventually carry out the exercises concentrically. Eccentric work may also be found useful during rehabilitation from injury.

However, there are some difficulties. Most weight-training equipment is designed for concentric work and eccentric exercises may not be easy to organise. In these circumstances lowering very heavy weights may be somewhat hazardous. Eccentric weight training is not a universal answer to all strength-development problems, but it has a number of advantages and athletes and coaches should be aware of its effects and possibilities.

Beginning a weight-training programme
1. A satisfactory level of health and general fitness is necessary before beginning any intensive training programme. Weight-lifting produces considerable stress on ligaments, and an increase in internal pressure in the abdomen and thorax also occurs. This is reversed as soon as the lift is over but it may cause problems in anyone with an abdominal weakness, such as a scar as the result of a recent operation, or a tendency to hernia. It is also undesirable in those with high blood pressure and some types of cardiac disease.

2. When the individual has acquired a satisfactory level of general fitness he should select the lifts he wishes to perform. The choice is dictated by the muscle groups which are to be developed. Any postural defects should also be taken into account. He should next learn the lifts and how to handle weights with safety. This step is crucial or the consequences may be unfortunate.

3. The programme should begin with high repetitions of lifts with reasonably light weights. There should be two, or preferably three, training sessions per week. The individual should select a weight that he can raise 20 times with a particular lift. He should then do the same for all the other lifts in the programme. At the first training session he should perform 10 to 15 consecutive repetitions of each exercise, resting for a few minutes between each. If no undue soreness results the next day, the duration of the sessions can be gradually increased over the next few weeks. The number of repetitions in each set should be increased to 20. The number of sets should then be raised from one to two and eventually from two to three. When the number of sets is more than one, a set of each exercise should normally be performed before going on to the second set of the first exercise. After three or four weeks the individual should be performing three sets of 15 repetitions of each exercise in his programme.

4. If very high levels of strength are required, the individual should now be in a position to begin a more strenuous programme. The 6 R.M. should be established for each exercise by finding the maximum

Fig. 4.2 Constant resistance strength training using a weight-training machine and free weights. The third photograph illustrates that a large number of different muscle groups are involved in many free-weight exercises.

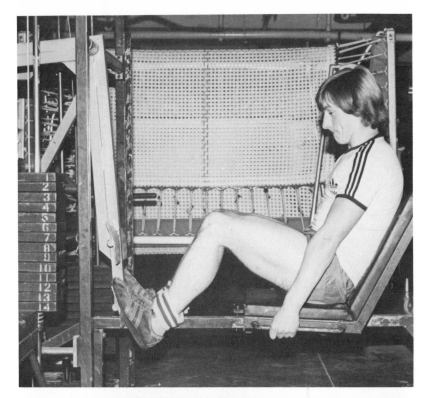

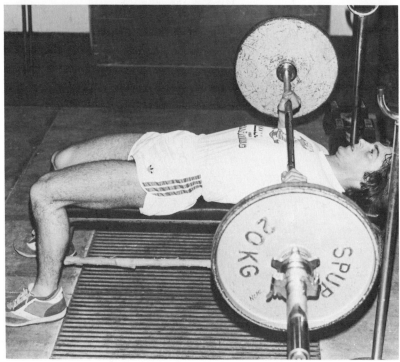

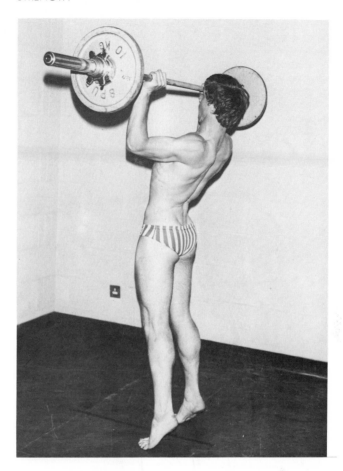

weight that can be lifted six times. The intensive programme should then begin with one set of each lift. Each set should consist of six repetitions with the 6 R.M. weight. If there are no ill-effects the number of sets can gradually be increased from one to three. As strength increases it will become possible to perform more than six repetitions of a particular exercise with the initial weight. When 10 are possible the weight should be increased so that the current 6 R.M. weight is again used (see Fig. 3.3).

With intensive weight programmes it is sometimes recommended that the three sets of a particular exercise should be completed before going on to the first set of the next exercise. Exercises which involve the largest muscle groups should be performed first. The above programme provides a gentle introduction to weight training. Younger individuals who are already used to training may be able to omit step 3.

Some coaches suggest that more than six repetitions are necessary to produce maximum strength increases in certain muscle groups, e.g. the calves and the abdominals. Twelve to fifteen repetions are often rec-

Fig. 4.3 A basic weight-training programme: (1) squat; (2) bent arm pull-over; (3) back hyper-extension; (4) military press; (5) arm curl; (6) dips with weights; (7) calf raiser; (8) abdominal leg raisers.

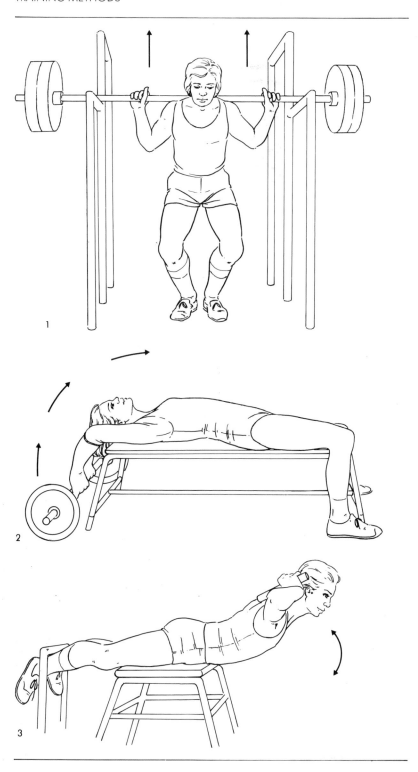

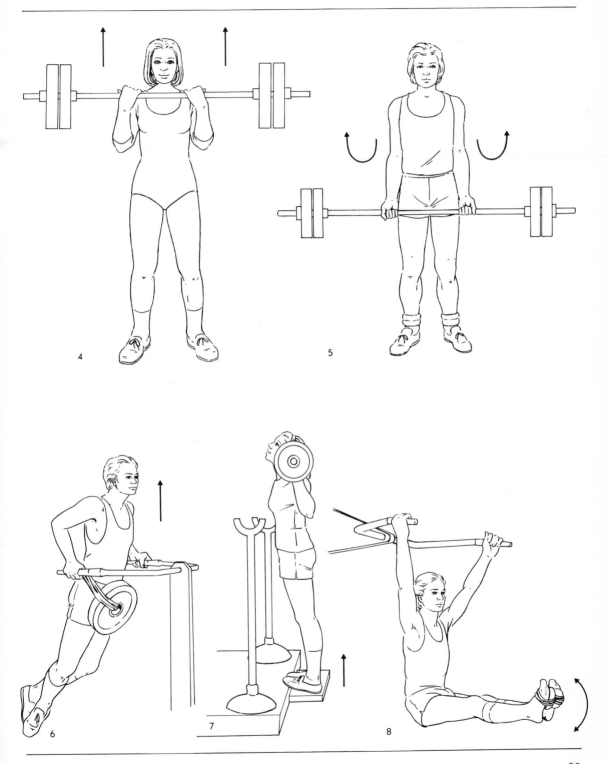

4

5

6

7

8

ommended. This matter does not appear to have been systematically investigated in any controlled study.

It has generally been found that weight training leads to an increase in the speed of movement (Zorbas and Karpovich 1951; Masley *et al.* 1953; Clarke and Henry 1961). Some authors report increases in motor performance on items such as the 50 yard dash (Chui 1950; Berger 1963) but this is not a universal finding (e.g. Dintiman 1964).

Some authors advocate the use of fast work with light weights as a means of increasing speed or power output. There seem to be no formal studies of this method of training. In a pilot investigation by the author, a group of subjects alternated normal weight-lifting with fast work using three-quarters of the normal resistance. This did appear to result in an increase in the power output available at high speed.

ISOMETRIC TRAINING

Isometric contractions can be used to improve strength. The normal training procedure consists of a series of short maximum contractions against the resistance of an immovable object or the opposite limb exercising in the same way. It is also possible to use contractions in antagonist muscles to resist those of the protagonists, e.g. simultaneous contraction of the biceps and triceps, or the quads and hamstrings. The resistance prevents movement and, because of this, maximum tension may be produced. In 1953 Hettinger and Müller suggested that one contraction of two-thirds maximum held for 6 seconds was all that was needed for optimal improvements in strength. It now appears that this is too little. If maximum gains are required it is probably better to use 5–10 maximal contractions, held for about 5 seconds each, training for five days per week (Müller and Rohmert 1963). One training session every two weeks is unlikely to produce any significant improvement, but one session per week may give 40 per cent of the improvement produced by daily training.

As with other types of training there are often variations in the response. Less frequently used muscles tend to respond most rapidly and gains may be slower in women and older individuals (Müller 1959). There are also individual variations. In two fairly large-scale studies about 20 per cent of the subjects demonstrated no gains at all (Hislop 1963; Morehouse 1967). The reasons for this are not clear, but in any case the effect is not confined to isometric training.

Isometric strength is to some extent specific to the joint angle employed during contraction. For a general improvement in strength, contractions at three different joint angles are recommended. This is most easily achieved in the type of training where the protagonist muscles are used to resist the contractions of the antagonists.

In organising an isometric programme the individual should first select the muscle groups that are to be trained. Using protagonist–antagonist contractions, each pair of muscle groups should be exercised near the middle of its normal range of movement. Begin with two or three maximum contractions. On subsequent days raise this to five, then six. At the fourth or fifth session work at other joint angles should begin. Start with three maximum contractions of each pair of muscle groups at the same joint angle as before. Follow this with three contractions near the maximum of each joint angle, then three more near the minimum. During subsequent sessions the number of contractions at each angle can be raised to five or more.

Isometric training generally produces significant increases in static strength. Dynamic strength is also increased but probably to a lesser degree (Rasch 1971). Some studies suggest that gains in static strength are equal to or greater than those achieved through an equivalent amount of dynamic work (Mathews and Kruse 1957; Rasch 1971). In a recent study Komi et al. (1978) have shown that isometric training produces increases in muscular endurance and also increases the concentrations of the enzymes hexokinase, malate dehydrogenase and succinate dehydrogenase in the trained muscles.

Absolutely no equipment is needed for a programme of isometric exercise. This appears to be its chief advantage. If equipment is available some form of weight training will probably produce improvements that are more specific to most kinds of sport. The static contraction of muscles tends to become boring rather quickly and it is difficult to detect improvements because no weights are being moved. A considerable rise in blood pressure may occur during the course of an isometric contraction. This is reversed when the tension is released but may be hazardous for older individuals or those suffering from hypertension. Despite these disadvantages isometric training may fulfil a useful function for individuals whose opportunity for other kinds of training is limited.

VARIABLE RESISTANCE TRAINING

The usual form of weight-lifting fails to produce maximum muscle tension throughout the whole range of movement, even if the weight lifted is the 1 Repetition Maximum. This occurs because of changes in the length of body lever-arms and because of the length-tension relationship of skeletal muscle. The situation was considered in detail in Chapter 2. It results in the muscle being maximally stressed only at one particular joint angle. In an attempt to stress the muscle maximally at all possible joint angles, training machines have been produced which produce *variable resistance*. This is achieved by connecting the limb to the weight through the mechanism of a cam. Examples of such machines are illustrated in Fig. 4.5.

The mechanics of each individual body movement is different and a separate machine is required for each type of movement.

Variable resistance training is relatively new and there have been few independent studies of the method. Peterson (1975) demonstrated significant increases in strength when subjects were tested on the same machine as was used for training. Pipes (1978) has carried out a comparison of a variable resistance programme with an equal amount of

Fig. 4.4 Isometric strength training. Resistance is provided by a wooden strut, muscle contraction in the opposite limb, and a belt. Note the marked distension of the arm veins illustrated in the first two photographs.

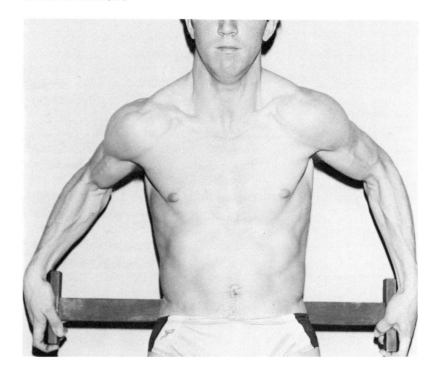

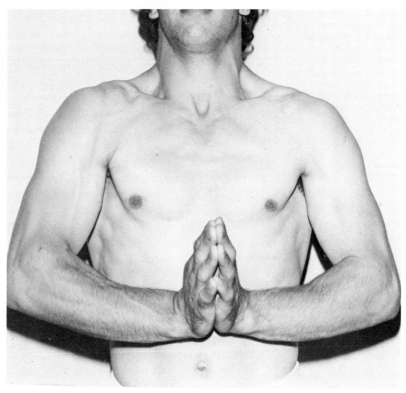

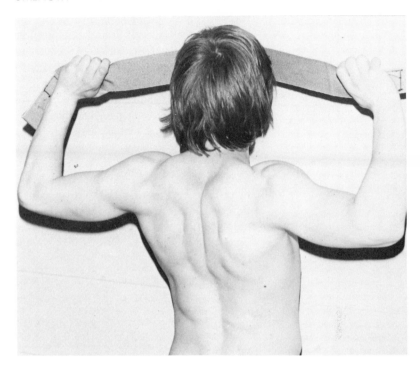

Fig. 4.5 Examples of variable resistance training machines. (Courtesy Nautilus Industries, Florida, USA.)

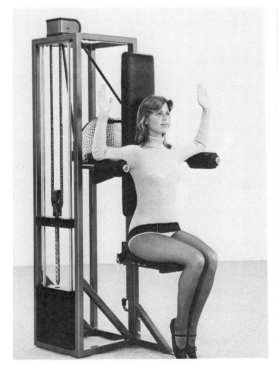

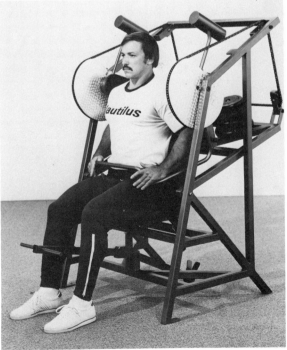

training on a normal weight-training machine (constant resistance). After 10 weeks it was found that both machines produced significant increases in strength. Subjects who trained on the variable resistance machine were significantly stronger than the constant resistance group when tested on the variable resistance machine; but subjects trained on the constant resistance machine were significantly stronger when tested on the constant resistance machine. Both groups had similar gains in fat-free weight and similar losses in body fat and skinfold thicknesses. These results suggest that both types of training produce similar changes in body composition. An example of the strength changes is given in Fig. 4.6. They are an excellent example of the concept of specificity. They show that the two types of training produce increases in different kinds of strength. The full extent of the changes are apparent only when the subject is tested with the same type of contraction as was used during training.

Fig. 4.6 Increases in leg-press strength following 10 weeks of weight training, three days per week. At each session three sets of eight repetitions were performed at 75 per cent of the 1 R.M. (Data from Pipes 1978).

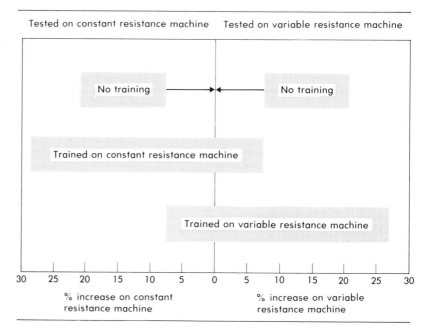

ACCOMMODATING RESISTANCE TRAINING (ISOKINETIC TRAINING)

In Chapter 2 it was noted that the force developed by a muscle is influenced by the speed of contraction. The ability to produce great force at low speed does not necessarily mean that the same will be true at higher speeds. Since many athletic activities require muscles to contract quickly, a type of training has been devised which allows rapid motion throughout the whole range of particular movements. When a weight is used as a resistance for training the speed of movement is generally lower at the start of motion because of the effects of inertia. There are

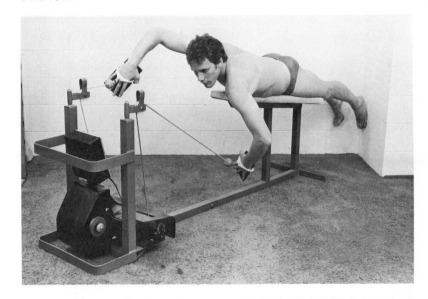

Fig. 4.7 Isokinetic strength-training devices. *Top*: swim-bench. *Bottom*: leaper. (Courtesy Mini Gym, USA.)

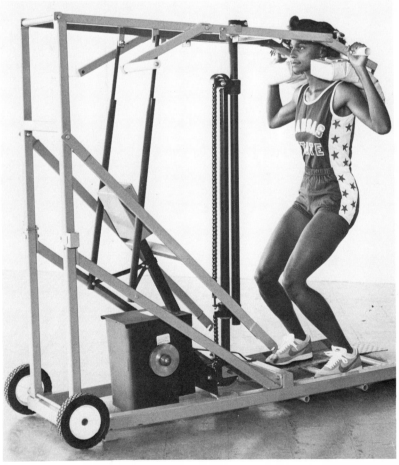

also variations due to changes in the effective force developed by the muscles. Isokinetic training devices are designed so that the resistance varies, or *accommodates*, allowing the movement to occur at constant speed. Some machines allow different speeds of movement to be selected. Examples of isokinetic training devices are shown in Fig. 4.7. The more elaborate machines are very expensive and often require ancillary equipment for different types of exercise. Rope friction devices are sometimes sold as isokinetic exercisers but little independent data is available on their effectiveness.

Fig. 4.8 Changes in strength at various speeds of limb movement following training on an isokinetic machine. Strength increased at and below the training speed but not at higher speeds. (Data from Lesmes *et al.* 1978a.)

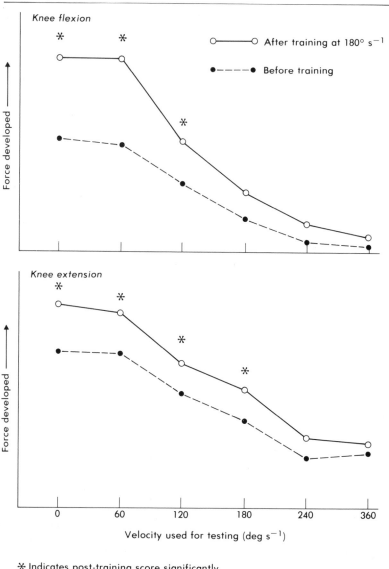

* Indicates post-training score significantly different from pre-training score

The results of a recent investigation into isokinetic training are summarised in Fig. 4.8. This study indicates that isokinetic training at a speed of 180° per second increased strength at this and lower speeds. There was no increase in strength at velocities higher than the training speed. The subjects trained four days per week for seven weeks and used either 10 × 6 s or 2 × 30 s work bouts per session. There were no significant differences in strength gains between these two procedures and both resulted in an increase in muscle phosphofructokinase concentration (Costill *et al*. 1979a). In an earlier study Pipes and Wilmore (1975) compared the effects of low-speed isokinetic training, high-speed isokinetic training and constant resistance weight training. Part of the results are summarised in Fig. 4.9.

The data again suggest that strength is increased at and below the training speed, but that low-speed training has little if any effect upon strength at high speeds of movement. Pipes and Wilmore also found that their isokinetic training improved performance in five motor performance tasks and produced larger changes in isometric strength than the constant resistance programme. Thistle *et al*. (1967) have also reported good results with an isokinetic training programme.

Fig. 4.9 Changes in leg-press strength following three different kinds of training: constant resistance, low-speed isokinetic, high-speed isokinetic. (Data from Pipes and Wilmore, 1975.)

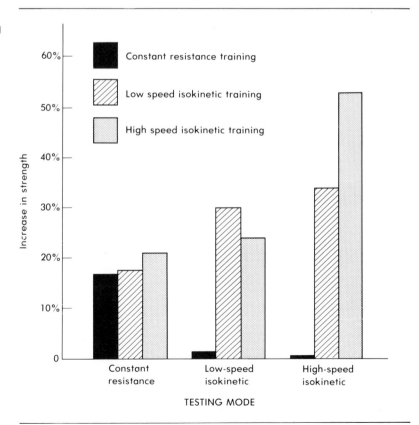

TRAINING WITH SPRING EXERCISERS

Springs are used as a resistance for strength training in the equipment illustrated in Fig. 4.10. Such devices are cheap and easily portable and are capable of producing increases in strength and muscle bulk. However, some manufacturers make excessively optimistic claims for this type of product. A direct comparison with other methods of training is not possible because no independent assessments of the effectiveness of spring exercisers are known. Such devices would appear to have a number of physiological and mechanical disadvantages. For example, the resistance offered is proportional to the degree of extension or compression of the spring. This is not an ideal arrangement for strength training as the force available from the majority of body-levers varies in a different way. It would suggest that other methods of strength training ought to produce changes in strength of greater benefit to the sportsman; but such devices should not be overlooked if other methods of training are not available.

When a spring exerciser is used for strength training a resistance should be selected which just allows between 5 and 10 repetitions of a particular exercise. As soon as more become possible further springs should be added so that the maximum is again between 5 and 10 repetitions. For all-round muscular development a range of several exercises is required. It is best to begin with one set of each, gradually working up to a maximum of three.

Training against body-weight resistance

Body-weight resistance is used for strength training in such exercises as push-ups, pull-ups, dips, trunk curls, leg lifts and back raisers. The range of muscles that can be developed is more limited than when weights or other devices are employed. Another problem is the difficulty in producing a satisfactory degree of overload. If the level is too low many repetitions are possible and gains in strength are low or non-existent. It is often possible to produce more overload by having the subject perform the exercise on an incline or by carrying extra weight.

The gains in strength are likely to be greatest when the overload is such that only 6–12 repetitions can be performed. As soon as more become possible the activity should be made more difficult. There are limitations as to how far this can be carried, and it is unlikely that extremely high levels of strength will be achieved. Useful gains are possible and the method should not be overlooked when no other is available.

PHYSIOLOGICAL CHANGES ACCOMPANYING INCREASES IN STRENGTH

Muscle hypertrophy is not an invariable consequence of training programmes that result in an increase in strength. For example, MacDougall *et al.* (1980) found no change in the fibre area of one subject whose strength increased by 143 per cent. There must, therefore, be

Fig. 4.10 Strength training devices based on springs.

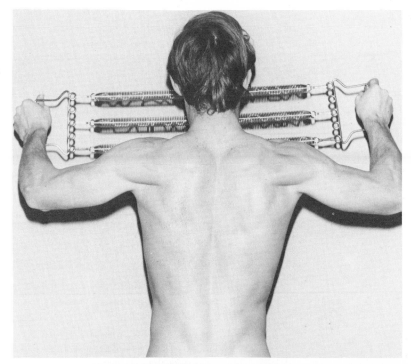

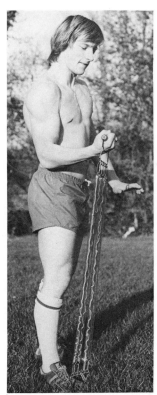

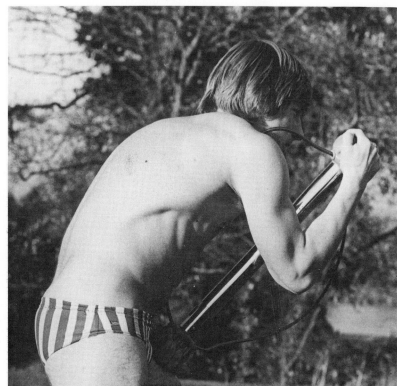

other changes in muscle following strength training. Neural adaption has been suggested (Lesmes *et al.* 1978a) and training probably increases the ability to synchronise motor units. There are also biochemical effects. MacDougall *et al.* (1977) found increases in muscle ATP and creatin phosphate after weight training. This presumably gives the muscle a greater capacity for aerobic work. Costill *et al.* (1979a) have noted an increase in the concentration of some of the enzymes of glycolysis, particularly phosphofructokinase.

An increase in muscular endurance accompanies high-intensity strength training. There seems little evidence to support the idea that work of lower intensity, with more repetitions, favours the development of muscular endurance (Clarke and Stull 1970; Stull and Clarke 1970). Costill *et al.* (1979a) found that training with ten 6 second work bouts had the same effect on endurance as a programme of two 30 second bouts.

STRENGTH TRAINING—SUMMARY AND CONCLUSIONS

All the previously described methods are capable of producing increases in strength. Isokinetic methods appear particularly attractive because of the reported rate of gain in the increase in strength at high speeds of contraction. However, it is difficult to come to firm conclusions with the data at present available. Many of the more esoteric training devices have a rather limited circulation and there is a lack of comparative information from independent sources. Constant resistance methods are more widely available and provide a useful basis of general strength. The simpler methods of training should not be overlooked if more elaborate procedures are not available.

For most athletes the important question is: '*Which method produces the greatest increase in performance?*' The literature on strength training fails to give an answer. This is not particularly surprising since most activities have different requirements. Some involve slow, almost isometric contractions, while others require extremely rapid motion against negligible resistance. It is clear that strength varies with the method of measurement. A training procedure would be expected to produce the best results under conditions similar to those occurring in the training process. Thus there is much to be said for forms of training that simulate the competitive activity.

The extent to which a general increase in strength can later be incorporated into a specific activity is not yet clear. Low-speed methods of strength training do not appear to increase the force that can be exerted at high speed, but they do result in increases in muscle bulk. Perhaps the athlete can learn to employ this tissue at higher speeds through skill training at a later date. This has yet to be determined.

ENDURANCE

In Chapter 2 'endurance' was defined as *the ability to continue to exercise at the highest possible work rate.* We saw that it is not particularly difficult to exercise for a long period of time. Problems arise only when one attempts to do so at a high rate of working. This situation arises because the body has several different mechanisms that provide energy for muscular contraction. The most powerful mechanisms are exhausted quickly and the individual must then rely on others which last longer but provide energy at a much lower rate. The characteristics of the principle methods of energy production are summarised in Fig. 4.11.

In order to improve endurance it is necessary to increase either the total capacity or the maximum output of the appropriate energy sources. The ones that are used in a particular situation depend upon a number of factors. The duration and intensity of the activity are primary considerations, but the characteristics of the athlete, including his state of training, also have an important influence.

Endurance is important only when the energy expenditure of an activity is high in relation to its duration. The energy for a very brief activity – e.g. an isolated jump or throw – can be provided from the muscle stores of ATP and creatin phosphate. In a sprint lasting 10–30 seconds the lactic acid mechanism is also used. If the activity involves 30 minutes of heavy work, 95 per cent of the energy comes from the oxidation of carbohydrates. In extremely protracted activities most of the energy is derived from fats.

It is more difficult to determine the major energy source in an intermittent activity. A footballer will use the same mechanisms as a sprinter during a short burst of speed that lasts a few seconds, but he will rely on aerobic processes for the lower level activity that occurs during most of the match. In one investigation into the activity pattern in the game of rugby it was found that more than 50 per cent of the action lasted between 5 and 10 seconds and only about 5 per cent went on for longer than 30 seconds (Williams, 1976). The 80 minute game consisted of only 27 minutes of actual play, which could be divided into 140 separate pieces of action. Of these, 120 lasted for no more than 15 seconds. Differences in the activity pattern of players in different positions were noted. Half the running done by the backs was at top speed while only one-third of that done by the forwards came into the same category. The demands of other sports will certainly be different and there will also be variations within a particular game and from individual to individual. It is impossible to make generalisations and the team coach must attempt to establish the activity pattern of his own players.

VARIOUS TYPES OF ENDURANCE

When planning a training programme it is useful to distinguish several different kinds of endurance. These stem both from the physiological energy sources and the way that they are employed during exercise. Their main characteristics are summarised in Table 4.3.

It is misleading to view endurance solely as a function of energy sources. Other important factors include the type of activity, the

Fig. 4.11 The four principal mechanisms that provide energy for muscular contraction. From: (a) high energy phosphate compounds, (b) production of lactic acid, (c) muscle glycogen (d) other carbohydrates and fats. The symbols E_1 to E_5 denote different sets of enzymes.

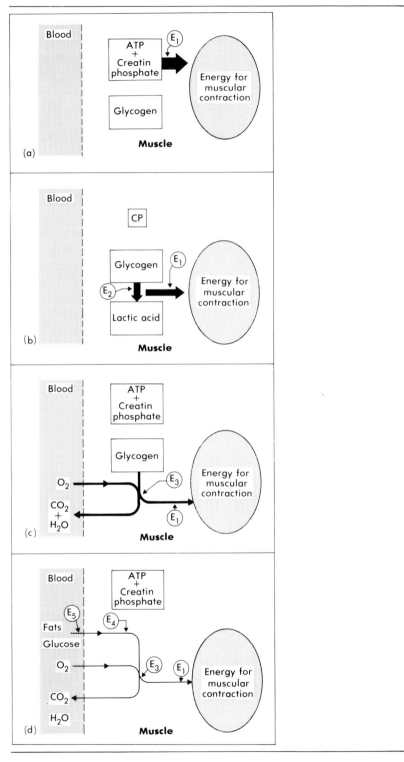

Type	A feature of	Example	Primary energy sources
Local muscular endurance (anaerobic)	Intensive activities of short duration usually involving small groups of muscles	Continuous weight-lifting	ATP and creatin phosphate; production of lactic acid.
Speed endurance Power endurance (anaerobic)	Intensive activities occurring at high speed and lasting for a few seconds	Short sprints	ATP and creatin phosphate (and possibly the production of lactic acid)
Lactic endurance (anaerobic)	Intensive activities lasting from 30 seconds to a few minutes	800 m running	Conversion of muscle glycogen into lactic acid
Local aerobic endurance	Strenuous activities involving small muscle groups that last for several minutes	Arm exercise of long duration, e.g. kayaking	Oxidation of muscle glycogen
Aerobic	Strenuous activities which last for several minutes in which large muscle groups are involved	Running, swimming, cycling, etc.	Oxidation of muscle glycogen
Long-term endurance	Activities which last more than 1 hour	Marathon, long-distance cycling, etc.	Oxidation of fats, etc.

Table 4.3 Characteristics of different types of endurance

efficiency with which it is executed, the determination of the athlete and his general physical condition. It is also a mistake to suppose that each energy source works in isolation from the others. They do not. In almost all kinds of exercise more than one type of endurance is employed and the different mechanisms are interdependent. But training can be made more effective if steps are taken to emphasise the types of endurance that are particularly relevant to the individual sportsman. Some of the assessment procedures discussed in Chapter 5 may be useful in this context.

LOCAL ANAEROBIC ENDURANCE

This is a feature of intensive activities, usually involving relatively small muscle groups. A prolonged contraction, or short repeated ones, depletes the stores of ATP and creatin phosphate, and lactic acid is then produced. This accumulates and eventually prevents the exercise being continued. This type of endurance is often known simply as *local muscular*. It is improved by strength training and other forms of intensive resistance exercise; the muscle stores of ATP and creatin phosphate are increased as a result (McDougall *et al.* 1977) and this presumably delays the accumulation of lactic acid. It seems that a few repetitions of very heavy lifts are as effective as a greater number with lighter weights provided that the total work done is the same in each case (De Lateur *et al.* 1968).

The increase in endurance is specific to the muscle groups trained so that general training programmes are ineffective. Brief periods of very intensive work are required; work with weights is ideal.

SPEED OR POWER ENDURANCE

This is similar to the previous kind of endurance except that muscular contraction occurs at high speed and usually involves large muscle groups. During very brief activities like the shot-put, power output is limited by neuromuscular considerations, not by endurance. For this type of activity high-speed isokinetic strength training is recommended. Depletion of the high-energy phosphate compounds in muscle will lead to a reduction in speed at the end of a 100 m sprint and will have a detrimental effect on performance in races up to 1,500 m. This type of endurance is also important in most team games. It can be improved by short, intensive work-outs, such as 60 second runs up a slight incline and 6 second dashes up a 44 per cent slope, followed by full recovery. After six weeks of such training, four times per week, Houston and Thomson (1977) noted a 15 per cent increase in muscle ATP concentration and a 17 per cent increase in the time for an anaerobic treadmill run. The capacity for lactate production was also increased. This type of endurance is important in many sports. In those which involve activities other than running it should be developed by short, intensive bouts of the appropriate activity, performed against additional resistance. These should be followed by a full recovery. Strength training on the appropriate muscles, especially high-speed work, is also beneficial.

LACTIC ENDURANCE

During intensive activities lasting from 15 seconds to a minute or so, a great deal of the energy is derived from the conversion of muscle glycogen into lactic acid. The rate of conversion depends upon the activity of certain key enzymes and the concentration of glycogen in muscle. Training leads to an increase in the rate of lactate production so that a greater intensity of effort is possible. This allows the 400 metre runner to go faster up the final straight. The total capacity for lactate production is also increased so that more high-intensity activity is possible. An untrained individual would have to run one lap of the 800 metres aerobically, and thus at a slow rate. A well-conditioned runner can just about manage this distance anaerobically and so can move at a much higher speed. Training also increases the athlete's tolerance to lactic acid and increases the rate at which this substance is removed.

There is a good deal of overlap between the methods of training for lactic, power and aerobic endurance. Both short-intensive work, followed by a full recovery, and long-continuous work are effective in untrained individuals, but the situation may be different in those who are already partially conditioned. It is possible that long-duration training may lead to a reduction in the maximum rate of lactic acid production. This was discussed on pages 39 and 40. In those sports where the period of activity lasts between 1 and 10 minutes, high-intensity training seems preferable. Unfavourable changes may occur if only low-intensity work is undertaken during part of the year. It seems that lactic endurance takes longer to develop than some other kinds. High-intensity training should be started early and continued for several months.

Sportsmen competing in longer events should not forget that the anaerobic energy sources are available to them on a 'once per race' basis, as illustrated in Fig. 4.12. This energy can make a significant contribution to performance. In this example anaerobic sources are shown to be equivalent to 9 litres of oxygen, but the actual quantity can vary between approximately 6 and 12 litres, depending upon several factors including the state of anaerobic training.

Fig. 4.12 The utilisation of anaerobic energy sources during exercise of long duration. *Top*: the energy available to a well-trained athlete from anaerobic and aerobic sources is shown. The athlete can use 5 litres of oxygen per minute and in addition has anaerobic sources equivalent to 9 litres of oxygen. *Bottom*: during a race lasting 4 minutes the athlete can take in 20 litres of oxygen. Anaerobic sources provide additional energy equivalent to another 9 litres. Thus the total rate of energy expenditure is equivalent to 7.25 litres of oxygen per minute (left). It is more usual for the greater part of the anaerobic sources to be utilised at the end of the race (right).

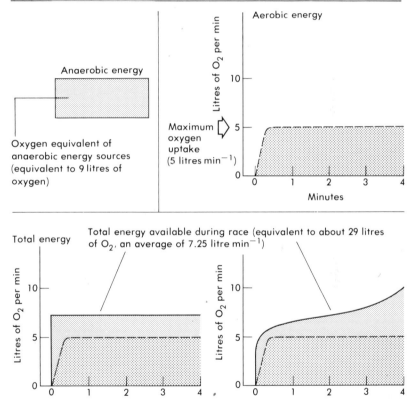

LOCAL AEROBIC ENDURANCE

Occasionally small muscle groups are required to work hard for an extended period of time. The situation occurs in kayaking and similar sports where most of the work is done with the arms. Energy production seems to be limited by the muscle's ability to extract oxygen from blood, not by the cardiovascular system (Prendergast 1979). Training should thus concentrate on the muscle groups concerned rather than the central circulation. Although the topic has not been widely studied, a number of points emerge.

Although strength training may be a valuable part of preparation for this type of activity it is not likely to increase local aerobic endurance. Less intensive effort is necessary, carried out over a much longer period. With this type of work the optimum training intensity is very difficult to establish; neither heart rate nor oxygen uptake are reliable guides. An intensity that can just be managed for five minute periods is suggested. Interval-type work on the muscles concerned can also be used.

AEROBIC ENDURANCE

Aerobic endurance has received considerably more attention from researchers than any other type and a later section is devoted to a review of this work. It is often referred to simply as *endurance*, a term that to some people is synonymous with *physical fitness*.

Aerobic processes provide the energy for activities of long duration and aerobic endurance is important for any continuous exercise that lasts for more than a minute. It is also necessary in short, intermittent activities where the energy sources are primarily anaerobic. If aerobic endurance is inadequate, the production of lactic acid commences at an extremely low level of energy expenditure and causes premature fatigue. This is illustrated in Fig. 4.13.

Fig. 4.13 The threshold of anaerobic metabolism in a trained and an untrained individual. An arbitrary value of 4 mmole lactic acid per litre of blood has been selected as the 'anaerobic threshold'. The untrained subject reaches this value when his oxygen intake is about 60 per cent of his $\dot{V}_{O_2max}$, while in the trained subject the value is 85 per cent. *Inset*: the trained subject also has a greater $\dot{V}_{O_2max}$ so that the anaerobic threshold is not reached until he is consuming over 4 litres of oxygen per minute. In the untrained individual the threshold is reached when the oxygen intake is only half this value.

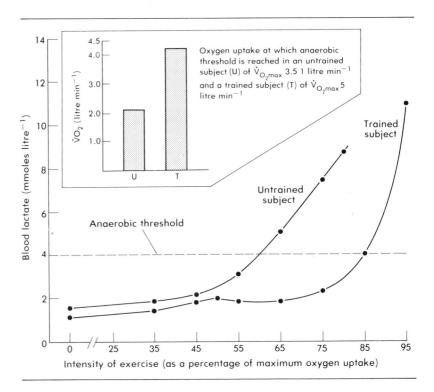

Aerobic fitness is also necessary to enable the athlete to undertake a warm-up which will raise body temperature and allow him to benefit fully from its effects.

LONG-TERM ENDURANCE

When maximum exertion lasts longer than an hour or so endurance is influenced by a different set of factors. The supply of fuels to muscle then limits energy production more than the availability of oxygen. Muscle glycogen stores are depleted and fats must be used as the primary fuel. There is also a possibility that glucose is manufactured from amino acids (Young *et al.* 1967; Rudermann 1975). Considerable biochemical adaptions are necessary to ensure an adequate supply of fuel during extended periods of exercise. These changes have been observed in athletes such as marathon runners (Scheel *et al.* 1979; Costill *et al.* 1979b; Lavine *et al.* 1980). Such effects include changes in the concentration of hormones in blood and enzymes in muscle.

During long races temperature regulation becomes a problem. Training produces adaptions which increase the contribution of sweating to heat loss. This preserves a greater proportion of the cardiac output for use by the working muscles. Training for long-term endurance has not been as extensively studied as some other kinds, but the evidence available suggests that long-duration training is necessary to bring about the adaptions described above.

REVIEW OF STUDIES OF AEROBIC TRAINING

Published studies in this area are numerous and a good deal is now known about the variables which influence aerobic fitness. In the majority of investigations the changes were followed by measuring the subject's maximum oxygen uptake. In a few cases other tests were used.

Endurance training is influenced by several variables including intensity, duration, frequency, placement, length, type and mode. These terms are also used in other forms of endurance training and are defined in Table 4.4.

Intensity
The training effect of exercise depends upon the amount of stress imposed upon the relevant part of the body. For this reason it is usual to quantify the intensity of aerobic training in terms of the percentage of maximum oxygen uptake used or the effect upon the heart rate. The latter is much easier to measure in a practical training situation. Since there are variations in the resting heart rate of different individuals the percentage of *heart-rate reserve* that is used in the exercise gives a better indication of intensity. Heart-rate reserve is the difference between the individual's maximum and resting heart rates, as illustrated in Fig. 4.14.

Davis and Convertius (1975) found that the percentage of heart-rate reserve used during exercise was highly related to the percentage of

Table 4.4 Terms used to quantify programmes of endurance training

Term	Meaning	Example
Intensity	The severity or degree of overload produced. Usually measured in terms of the effect upon cardiorespiratory variables	The heart rate produced by the exercise or the % of $\dot{V}_{O_2\text{max}}$ used
Duration	The length of each training session	
Frequency	The number of training sessions per week	Three per week
Placement	The distribution of training sessions in the week	Monday, Tuesday and Wednesday *or* Monday, Wednesday and Friday
Length	The number of weeks of training	
Type	Whether continuous or interval	
Mode	The type of exercise	Swimming, running or cycling

Fig. 4.14 The heart-rate reserve and its relationship to resting and maximum heart-rates.

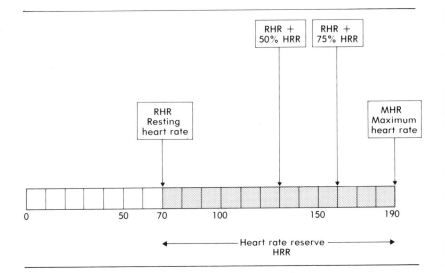

$\dot{V}_{O_2\text{max}}$. The relationship was closest when resting heart rate was measured after the subject had been standing still for 10 minutes. A number of authors have questioned the use of the above measures for determining the intensity of endurance training. The point at which anaerobic work begins (the anaerobic threshold) may be a better guide (see Kindermann *et al.* (1979) for further details). Such parameters are too difficult to measure to be of general use. Until other methods are developed the use of heart-rate reserve is recommended for training purposes.

The influence of intensity of training on gains in aerobic fitness has been studied more often than any other variable. Perhaps for this reason its effects are often overstated, especially in older books. Recent work suggests that although there is a minimum intensity of exercise below which no gains in aerobic fitness occur, once this has been reached the other variables are also important. The critical intensity is a level of stress greater than that which the subject normally experiences. Gains in endurance have been reported following exercise at between 120 and 135 beats per minute (Durnin *et al.* 1960; Glenhill and Eynon 1972; Kilbom 1971) and using 50 per cent of the heart-rate reserve (Kearne *et al.* 1976). With fitter subjects heart rates up to 150 beats per minute are required (Karnoven *et al.* 1957; Roskamm 1967). For very fit subjects even greater overload is necessary.

Duration

It has been established more recently that the duration of training also affects the increase in aerobic capacity. Greater gains occur during 20–30 minute periods of work than from 10 minute periods (Shephard 1968; Davies and Knibbs 1971). These authors concluded that the intensity of training was still a more important influence than duration. However, in the above investigations the subjects who exercised at the higher intensities did a greater amount of work. In four other studies the total work done by the subjects was held constant (Sharkey 1970; Kearne *et al.* 1976; Fox *et al.* 1977; Lesmes *et al.* 1978b). It was then found that there was no significant difference in the effects of increases in duration or intensity. Shire *et al.* (1977) found no difference in the effects of high-speed low-intensity training, and low-speed high-intensity exercise when the total work done was held constant.

Frequency

Several studies have found that training for only one day per week produced no improvement in aerobic fitness (Shephard 1968; Davies and Knibbs 1971; Jackson *et al.* 1968), but gains have been reported following programmes undertaken for two days per week (Pollock 1973) and three is usually recommended. It is not clear whether there is an advantage in training for more than three days per week. Some studies suggest that greater gains do occur (Pollock *et al.* 1969; Shephard, 1968); others come to the opposite conclusion (Jackson *et al.* 1968; Atomi *et al.* 1978). Training for five days per week may increase the risk of injury (Pollock *et al.* 1977).

Placement

One study has shown that the placement of tri-weekly training sessions is unimportant. Gains were as great when training took place on consecutive days as when it occurred on Monday, Wednesday and Friday (Moffatt *et al.* 1977).

Initial level of fitness

The initial level of fitness has an important influence on the rate of improvement. As with strength, those who begin at a low level tend to improve more rapidly and achieve the greatest gains. An extreme example is a group of post-coronary patients who trained for, and completed, a marathon. Their gains in $\dot{V}_{O_2\text{max}}$ averaged 57 per cent (Kavanagh *et al.* 1974). The gain for an average subject would be expected to be 10–20 per cent.

Age

In children aerobic capacity is determined primarily by considerations of size and it is not clear whether training has much effect. But it is important in the elderly. Although aerobic capacity declines with age, training produces similar percentage increase in individuals up to 80 years of age as it does in younger subjects.

Gender

The majority of training studies have been carried out on males but there are now a number of reports showing that women respond to endurance training in the same way as men (Kilbom, 1971, Cunningham *et al.* 1979; Atomi and Miyashita 1974, 1978; Smith and Stransky 1976; Kearne *et al.* 1976; Atomi *et al.* 1978; Lesmes *et al.* 1978b). Post-puberal females have a lower aerobic capacity than post-puberal males, but training appears to produce a similar percentage increase in both sexes.

Length

The majority of studies on endurance training show that gains in aerobic capacity are greatest during the first 4–8 weeks. Thereafter increases are small or non-existent. An example is given in Fig. 4.16 on page 116. It is obviously necessary to increase the training load as the programme proceeds and the subjects become fitter. But even then gains are slow after 6–8 weeks. This seems to be about the right length of programme to give team-game players at the start of the season. Longer periods of training are useful for endurance athletes but significant further increases in maximum oxygen uptake do not usually occur unless intensive training is continued for several months.

Mode – The specificity of endurance training

The mode of exercise employed in endurance training has an important effect upon the result. This is because a considerable proportion of the physiological changes that occur take place in the muscles that are exercised, rather than in the cardiovascular system. These changes were discussed in some detail in Chapter 2. This means that the increase in capacity for oxygen transport is, to a large extent, specific to the mode of exercise used during training. Two recent studies which illustrate this point are summarised in Fig. 4.15.

Swim-training was found to have no effect upon the maximum oxygen uptake measured while running, and running had only a small effect on the maximum oxygen uptake during swimming. The authors of these studies speculate as to whether running has a more general

Fig. 4.15 Increases in maximum oxygen uptake following swim training and run training. The values on the left were measured while the subjects were swimming; those on the right during running. (Data from Magel *et al.* 1975 and McArdle *et al.* 1978)

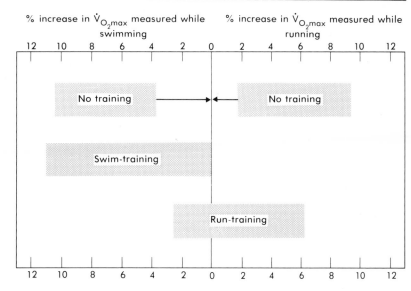

effect upon aerobic fitness than swimming. They consider that it may have, but do not rule out the possibility that the increase in swimming $\dot{V}_{O_2max}$ after run-training was due to a local training effect upon the leg muscles. Other investigations show that an athlete's maximum oxygen uptake is higher during the activity for which he has trained than it is when he runs on a treadmill (Strømme *et al.* 1977). Bouchard *et al.* (1979) measured the $\dot{V}_{O_2max}$ of moderately active subjects while performing five different tasks. They found that the overall common variance between $\dot{V}_{O_2max}$ scores measured during different tasks was only about 50 per cent of the total variance. Other workers have reported similar results (Glassford *et al.* 1965; Bar-Or and Zwiren 1975). These studies indicate that the effects of aerobic training are highly specific to the activities undertaken. The muscles are just as much involved in the process of adaption as the central circulation. If the aim of the training is merely a non-specific improvement in general physical condition, perhaps for health reasons, then almost any form of continuous activity is capable of improving cardiovascular function. But if the objective is to improve endurance in a particular activity, the training should be as much like that activity as possible or the results will be disappointing.

Aerobic capacity is so specific that changes in the maximum oxygen uptake of the whole body may not be a good guide to increases in endurance in relation to a particular activity. Figure 4.16 shows changes in running speed and $\dot{V}_{O_2max}$ of two groups who trained for 8 weeks. In the previously untrained group the change in $\dot{V}_{O_2max}$ during the first 4 weeks (+ 9 per cent) closely paralleled that in running speed (+ 8 per cent). But after 4 weeks, and in the previously trained group, running

Fig. 4.16 Changes in $\dot{V}_{O_2max}$, and time over 880 yd and 2 miles following training. *Above:* for previously untrained individuals. *Below:* for previously trained subjects. In both groups running speed increased as the training proceeded. These changes did not parallel those occurring in $\dot{V}_{O_2max}$. In the previously trained group no change in $\dot{V}_{O_2max}$ occurred and in the previously untrained group it rose only during the first four weeks of training. (Data from Daniels *et al.* 1978b)

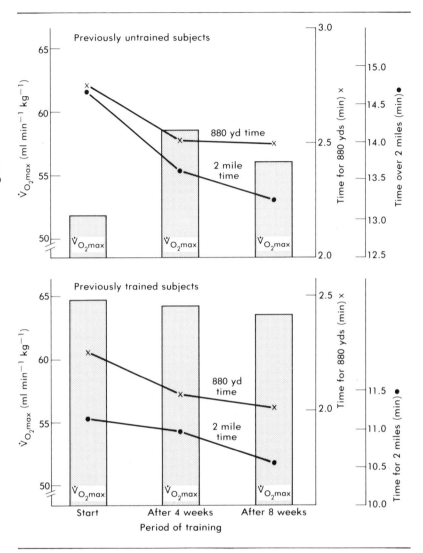

speed increased despite the fact that $\dot{V}_{O_2}$ remained approximately constant. The authors suggest that this may be due to local adaptions in the muscles concerned in running.

TYPES OF TRAINING – CONTINUOUS VS. INTERVAL

Most modes of exercise can be carried out either at a continuous, steady rate or as short bursts of intense activity separated by rest or more moderate exercise. The latter is known as *interval training*. The procedure allows more high-intensity work to be undertaken in a given period. This is possible because anaerobic energy sources are utilised which are replenished during the recovery phase of the training process. Interval work can be used to train for any of the types of endurance previously described by varying the duration and intensity of work undertaken during the exercise and rest periods. It might be expected that short, intensive work intervals followed by long periods of rest would tend to develop speed endurance while having less effect on aerobic capacity. Many books on interval training suggest that long work intervals develop aerobic capacity while intermediate ones of 400 to 800 metres have a particular effect on lactic endurance. Practical studies on the effects of training programmes do not always support these ideas and sometimes indicate that the differences between continuous and interval training are small.

One of the advantages claimed for interval training is its effect on lactic endurance. Some studies have shown that short periods of such training do increase this capacity (for example, Kilbom 1971; Eddy *et al.* 1977) but a number of others have failed to confirm this (Fox *et al.* 1977; Lesmes *et al.* 1978b; Cunningham *et al.* 1979). These were studies of short periods of training and, as mentioned earlier, it is possible that changes in the lactic acid system may require a longer period to develop. Also it is difficult to know how much energy an athlete has obtained from the production of lactic acid and this makes comparisons of different training methods difficult. Continuous exercise may be just as effective as interval training provided it is of sufficient intensity.

It would be expected that high-intensity interval training would be a more effective method of increasing power endurance than continuous running, but the difference has never been clearly demonstrated. Both methods are capable of increasing the concentration of ATP in muscle (Karlsson *et al.* 1972; Eriksson *et al.* 1973; Houston and Thomson 1977). However, no direct comparison of the two methods seems to have been made. Attempts to demonstrate an increase in anaerobic power out-put following interval training have not been successful (Fox *et al.* 1977; Houston and Thomson 1977). The test used in these studies involved less than a second of intense activity, and it is possible that a longer work period might have produced a different result. It seems likely that interval training needs to be very intense if it is to have effects different from those of ordinary running. Although the body adapts differently to different kinds of stress, it does not react to small changes. Intervals must be very short and intensive if they are to have a special effect and the additional resistance of sprinting up an incline may be necessary.

Continuous and interval training have a similar effect upon aerobic endurance. The changes in maximum oxygen uptake are the same with both types of training when the total work done by the subjects is equal (Pollock *et al.* 1975; Cunningham *et al.* 1979; Eddy *et al.* 1977). Continuous and interval training have also been shown to produce similar increases in leg speed (Ragg 1979).

Despite the lack of physiological differences between the two types of training there are often features which may be important. Interval training is more highly structured so that it is easier to control the training dosage, the combination of intensity and duration that produces the training effect. Conversely, interval work requires a greater amount of organisation and useful results are unlikely without some degree of planning and organisation. Interval training would seem to have advantages in the preparation for intermittent activities, like most team games. It is closer to the situation that actually occurs in many sports, and short intervals of high-speed movement are probably a better preparation for most team games than longer periods of slower work.

Continuous exercise is likely to be the best type of training for very long events. An increasing proportion of fats are oxidised as the duration of the activity increases. Long-duration training raises the proportion of fats utilised, so sparing muscle glycogen reserves (Paul and Holmes 1975). The concentration of enzymes involved in fatty acid oxidation is increased by this type of training (Hermansen et al. 1967; Mole and Holloszy 1970; Mole et al. 1971). This change does not occur with short, high-intensity training (Staudte et al. 1973). The body must also adapt to cope effectively with the dissipation of heat (Baum et al. 1976). This and several other necessary changes are likely to be brought about through long-duration training.

It is sometimes said that slow, long-duration exercise achieves greater capillarisation of muscle. There appear to be no studies which show that long-duration training is superior to other types in this respect.

ENDURANCE TRAINING BY THE CONTINUOUS METHOD

1. General effect on the cardiovascular system

Such a programme may be required by the sedentary adult who wishes to improve his general physical condition. Any type of exercise can be used as long as it involves large muscle groups and produces a heart rate in the range 120–150 beats per minute. It does not have to be particularly strenuous; gains in aerobic fitness have been reported using programmes of walking, running, skipping, cycling, swimming, callisthenics, squash and dancing (Durnin et al. 1960; Pollock et al. 1975; Wilmore et al. 1975; data from the author), but first ensure the individual is basically healthy and equipped with suitable footwear which is comfortable and well padded. A jogging programme suitable for this type of individual is given in Table 4.5. Training should occur about three times per week. A higher frequency may increase the risk of injury (Pollock et al. 1977).

2. Players of team games

At the start of training the jogging programme in Table 4.5 can be used, beginning about stage 10 and omitting the odd-numbered stages. A progression should then be made to short-distance interval work or Fartlek-type training. This should be carried out in 15–30 minute sessions, two or three times per week for 6–8 weeks.

Table 4.5 A progressive programme of jogging

Stage	Activity	Distance (miles)	Target time (min)
1	Walk	1	20
2	Walk	1½	30
3	Alternate: walk 660 yd, fast walk 220 yd.	1½	28½
4	Alternate: walk 440 yd, fast walk 440 yd.	1½	27
5	Alternate: walk 220 yd, fast walk 440 yd.	1½	25½
6	Fast walk	1½	24
7	Alternate: fast walk ⅜ mile, slow jog ⅛ mile	1½	22
8	Alternate: fast walk ¼ mile, slow jog ¼ mile	1½	20
9	Alternate: fast walk ⅛ mile, slow jog ⅜ mile	1½	18
10	Slow jog	1½	16
11	Slow jog	2	22
12	Slow jog	2	20
13	Alternate: slow jog ⅜ mile, jog ⅛ mile	2	19
14	Alternate: slow jog ¼ mile, jog ¼ mile	2	18
15	Alternate: slow jog ⅛ mile, jog ⅜ mile	2	17
16	Jog	2	16
17	Jog	2½	23
18	Jog	2½	20
19	Jog	3	27
20	Jog	3	24

3. Endurance athletes

Use the mode of activity employed in competition. It is difficult to give any other advice because there are so many variables and relatively few studies in the area. For 'middle distance' athletes it would seem sensible to spend about half the time training at the competitive distance with the other half equally divided between 'overdistance' and 'underdistance' work. These latter types of training should differ from the competitive distance by a factor of at least three times.

INTERVAL TRAINING

A description of the terms used in interval training is given in Table 4.6. A large number of variables can be manipulated in order to produce different types of programme.

The work interval should be selected first. This can be done either in terms of distance – the training distance – or time – the work interval. In the case of a track athlete it may be best to begin with a training distance close to that run in competition. When training for a game the distance should be selected to produce a work interval corresponding to the most common duration of intense activity. For most sports short training distances of 50–100 m are usually suitable.

It is now necessary to ensure the correct training intensity. This is done by adjusting the training time so that the training distance is covered at a suitable pace. The subject's heart rate at the end of the work interval is often used as a guide. One hundred and eighty beats per min-

Table 4.6 Terms used in interval training

Term	Meaning	Example
Work interval	Period during which intensive work is performed	Period during which 400 m is run
Relief interval	A period of rest or light work between work intervals	Rest, walking or slow running
Training mode	Type of activity undertaken	Running, swimming or cycling
Training distance	Distance covered in each work interval	400 m
Training time	Time for each work interval	60 s for each 400 m
Repetitions	Number of work intervals per set	Four work intervals of 400 m running
Set	A group of intervals	A set might consist of four repetitions of a 400 m run
Session	A group of sets of repetitions	A session might consist of two sets of four repetitions of a 400 m run
Work : relief ratio	Ratio of duration of work interval to duration of relief interval	1 : 2 means 60 s for each work interval and 120 s for each relief interval
Frequency of training	Number of training sessions per week	Three sessions per week

ute is often recommended for subjects under 30 years of age, 10 beats per minute less for every 10 years above this age. The heart rate should be determined by counting the pulse for 10 seconds and multiplying by 6 or by timing 30 beats with a stop-watch. Since the heart rate drops rapidly after the conclusion of a short interval, a longer count gives a low result. If the measurement of heart rates is impossible, training times can be estimated by adding between 10 and 20 per cent to the best time over the distance.

The next variable that needs to be considered is the duration of the relief interval. This must be long enough to allow regeneration of the ATP/creatin phosphate stores – 20-30 seconds is about the minimum time required. If the relief interval is too long the aerobic effects of the training will be reduced. Once again heart rate is a good guide. It should drop to about 150 beats per minute by the end of the relief interval. In most individuals the time for this drop is related to the length of the work interval. It is usually 2–3 times the duration of short work intervals, dropping to ½–¼ for much longer ones. Suggested ratios of work intervals: relief intervals are given in Table 4.7. These may be used as a guide if it is difficult to measure recovery heart rates. Longer relief intervals may be desirable in short-distance work, as discussed below.

The relief interval can consist of either complete rest or work of a lower intensity. If the training is for an activity where speed is of at least as much importance as endurance, then short, fast intervals should be used with relatively long relief intervals of complete rest. Try a work: relief ratio of 1 : 4 or extend the relief interval until the heart rate drops to 130 beats per minute.

In longer intervals of 0.5–2 minutes duration a significant proportion of the energy is derived from the production of lactic acid. It has been shown that lactic acid is removed more rapidly during moderate work than during complete rest. In one study it was found that athletes selected the optimum rate of working for themselves. Light activity is therefore the most suitable type of recovery for this sort of interval, the intensity being left to the individual. With even longer intervals there seems to be no convincing reason for preferring one type of recovery activity to the other. The mode should be determined by the individual's preference.

The other variables in interval training are: the number of intervals per session; the organisation of intervals into sets; and the training frequency. Some of these are considered in Table 4.7. The maximum number of intervals per session will determine the total distance covered. This varies from about 1½ miles for the shorter intervals up to about 2½ miles. These distances are about right for young individuals seeking to achieve quite rapid gains in endurance. The shorter intervals have been grouped into a series of sets. A longer relief interval should occur between sets to allow for the removal of lactic acid and other metabolites which gradually build up during the work intervals. The heart rate should be allowed to drop to about 120 beats per minute before the next set is started. The optimum training frequency would appear to be three times per week. A higher frequency is not all that

Table 4.7 Parameters of interval training programmes

Training distance (m)			Sets per training session	Maximum repetitions per set	Maximum repetitions per session	Work: relief ratio	Type of relief	Reputed to develop
Running	Swimming	Cycling						
50	–	100	10	5	50	1:3	Rest relief for	Speed, speed
100	25	300	6	4	24	or longer	running and swimming; light work in cycling	endurance, short-term endurance, ATP-CP system; also longer term endurance
200	50	500	4	4	20	1 : 2	Work relief.	Lactate
400	100	900	2 or 3	4	10		Exercising at half speed or whatever speed feels comfortable	endurance and aerobic endurance
800	200	1 mile	2 or 3	2	5–10	1 : 1	Either rest	Aerobic
1,200	400	2 miles	3 or 4	1	4–5	1 : 0.5	or work relief	endurance

likely to result in significantly greater gains but improvements will be slower if training occurs less often. Useful gains in aerobic endurance can be made in 6–8 weeks. After this, progress is much slower and very long periods of training are normally required for other significant gains. Short-term gains in endurance appear to be reversed equally quickly so that this type of training should be timed to end close to the start of the competitive season. Gains in anaerobic endurance may take longer to achieve, and this type of training should last for two or three months.

The training programme should be introduced gradually. The first two or three sessions might consist of easy running, before training times are determined. At the start of training the number of intervals per session should be one-third to one-half of the maximum intervals shown in Table 4.7. The number is then gradually increased over the first few sessions. Training should not produce exhaustion or undue soreness. Fitness is unlikely to improve if this occurs. The number of intervals must be adjusted so that a training overload is produced but exhaustion is avoided.

This section on interval training has been written with running as the exercise mode. The same principles can be applied equally to any other continuous activity such as swimming, cycling or rowing. Sportsmen requiring to develop power endurance should consider interval training with an increased resistance to movement. The training intensity should be high and the work intervals short – 5-10 seconds. Relief intervals must allow for complete recovery and should not be shorter than 1 minute.

OTHER FORMS OF ENDURANCE TRAINING

Fartlek training   A forerunner of interval training, the method involves alternate fast and slow running, often carried out over varied countryside. In pleasant districts the terrain may make this type of training attractive. Neither the work nor rest intervals are precisely controlled and the results will obviously depend upon the particular programme undertaken. Fartlek training is normally used to improved aerobic capacity. Hill-sprinting is sometimes included in the schedule, and this is likely to benefit anaerobic endurance.

Acceleration sprints   The individual begins at a slow pace and accelerates, eventually reaching top speed. He then decelerates and jogs or walks for a period before beginning the next acceleration. This type of training incorporates an element of warm-up and may be found a welcome change from other methods.

Hollow sprints   Two sprints separated by a period of jogging or walking.

OTHER ASPECTS OF FITNESS AND TYPES OF TRAINING

FLEXIBILITY

Flexibility is improved by stretching exercises. A selection of these is illustrated in Fig. 4.17. Stretching exercises should be performed slowly and the final position held for a few seconds. Jerky or ballistic movements are hazardous and may lead to injury. Static flexibility can often be increased dramatically by a few minutes of warm-up exercises. Stretching procedures should always be incorporated into the warm-up which precedes activities of a ballistic nature. They should also be used in conjunction with programmes of strength training otherwise a reduction in joint mobility may result.

Stretching exercises increase the range of movement of a joint but their effect on *ease* of movement is more obscure. It is not clear whether increasing the range of movement of the hip and leg joints makes for easier movement in an activity like sprinting. It would appear that other factors probably have a greater influence on the resistance to movement during a dynamic activity, but an increase in static flexibility will lessen the likelihood of muscle strain and may lead to the development of a more efficient running style. Ballistic flexibility exercises are sometimes undertaken by sprinters and throwers. This practice would appear potentially hazardous, the absence of normal resistance to motion increasing the likelihood of injury. Undesirable reflexes may also be developed during such activities.

SPEED (RUNNING SPEED)

The ability to run fast is strongly influenced by inate factors and the improvements possible through training are probably more limited than with most other aspects of fitness. Gains in speed are brought about as much through improvements in coordination and technique as by changes in measurable physiological variables. Correct sprinting style must be emphasised. There should be full flexion at the knee and hip with adequate stride length. A powerful arm action is important and 'rolling' at the shoulder should be avoided.

Speed is important in most team games and sprint work is often included in general training programmes. This is an effective method of improving speed. It develops the power output of appropriate muscle groups and helps to improve coordination. A good sprinting technique should be emphasised. For most team games the training distance should be kept short – between 10 and 30 yards is appropriate. A full recovery should be allowed after each run; speed training should not be incorporated into endurance work. Sprinting is best carried out at the beginning of the training session, following the warm-up.

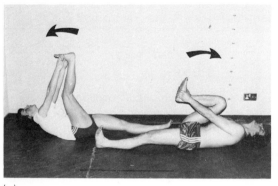

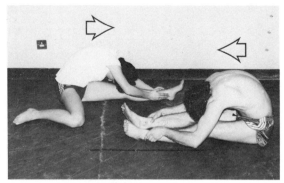

(a)

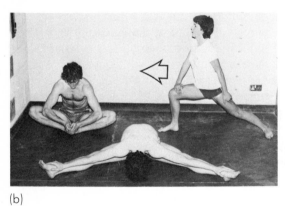

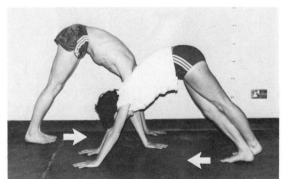

(b)

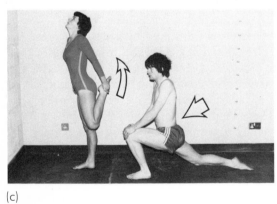

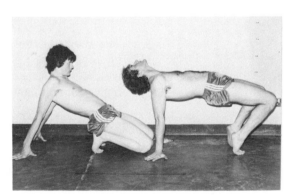

(c)

Fig. 4.17 Flexibility exercises: (a) for hamstrings, (b) for groin and calves, (c) for quads and (d–f) for the upper body.

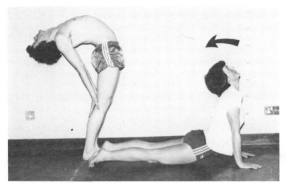
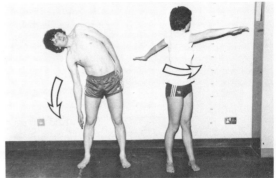

(d)

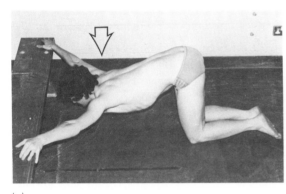
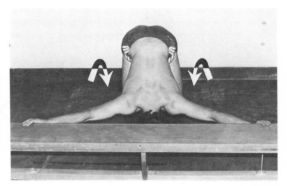

(e)

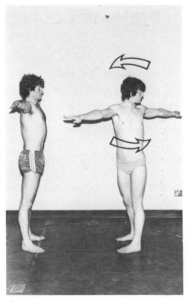
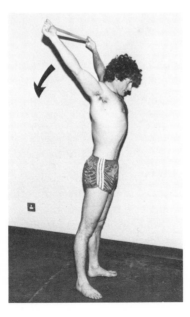
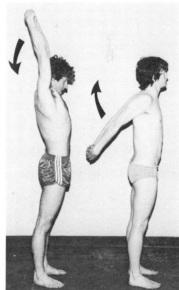

(f)

A second type of speed is also important – the ability to respond and move quickly when tired and under pressure in the middle of a match. This is a different skill from sprinting when fresh. It is appropriate to train for this aspect of fitness under conditions simulating those occurring in the game. However, this latter type of training should be kept separate from the acquisition of running speed which is a quite different skill.

The training methods used by sprinters are almost as diverse as cures for rheumatism. In some ways the two have a good deal in common. In contrast to the situation with strength and endurance there are no training methods for speed which have been shown to work universally. A wide variety of different approaches seems to produce favourable results in certain individuals. A number of these are summarised below.

1. Improve sprinting technique. This is probably the most certain method of increasing speed.

2. Decrease body weight by reduction of fat content. This will allow greater acceleration for a given level of dynamic strength. The reduction of excess fat on the thighs and legs is of particular importance

3. Develop appropriate muscle groups through strength training. Any type of strength training may be useful but fast work on an isokinetic machine is likely to be particularly beneficial. If isokinetic equipment is not available some coaches suggest that normal weight training should be followed by a period where rapid lifts are made using light weights ($\frac{1}{2}-\frac{3}{4}$ of the 6 RM).

4. Improve flexibility. Poor flexibility will mitigate against the development of a good sprinting technique and will increase the likelihood of injury.

5. Use an extended warm-up. A period of 15–20 minutes of heavy exercise – enough to produce sweating – will raise body temperature and increase power output. An adequate level of endurance is obviously a prerequisite.

6. Plyometrics or bounding exercises. These have been shown to have a favourable effect on sprinting speed (see p. 130).

7. Assisted running. This consists of sprinting down an incline. It has been successfully used by some athletes, and is probably an aid to the development of coordination at high speed. *Resisted running*, where the athlete sprints while being restained by a harness, is also used; presumably this acts as a stimulus to the development of leg power.

8. Arm work with a speed-ball. This consists of punching an object suspended so as to swing within a small arc; presumably it assists in the development of arm power or coordination.

INCREASING BODY WEIGHT – BODY-BUILDING

An increase in body weight is often an advantage to the athlete involved in such activities as throwing events and body contact sports. Provided that speed does not suffer, momentum is increased and this can be transferred to a throwing implement or opponent. Extra body weight will also help the individual absorb the momentum of other sportsmen in games like football and rugby, and the extra muscle protects the skeleton and aids joint stability. A programme which has been successfully used with experienced sportsmen is given in Table 4.8.

Individuals vary in their capacity to develop muscle. This may be related to somatotype or muscle-fibre composition, but even the 'slow-gainer' is capable of some muscle development if he persists with training.

Table 4.8 Advanced Weight Training Schedule (courtesy E.J.M. O'Sullivan)

Schedule A. Emphasis on the upper body

Exercise	Sets and repetitions	Main muscles developed	Part of body developed
Bench press	3 sets × 12 reps	Pectoralis and triceps	Chest and arms Shoulders
Dips	3 sets × 15 reps		
Bent arm pull-over	3 sets × 12 reps		
Flies	4 sets × 15 reps		
Dumb-bell press	4 sets × 12 reps	Deltoids	
Alternate dumb-bell curl	4 sets × 12 reps	Biceps	Arms and forearms
Reverse curls	4 sets × 12 reps	Forearm muscles	
Triceps extensions	4 sets × 12 reps	Triceps	
Concentrated dumb-bell curl	4 sets × 12 reps	Biceps	
Sit-ups	3 sets × 15 reps	Rectus abdominus	Abdominals
Hanging leg raises	3 sets × 15 reps		

Schedule B. Emphasis on the legs, back and abdomen

Exercise	Sets and repetitions	Main muscles developed	Part of body developed
Front squat	3 sets × 15 reps	Quads	Legs
Hamstring curl	3 sets × 15 reps	Hamstrings	
Calf raises	3 sets × 15 reps	Gastrocnemius	
T-bar row	3 sets × 12 reps	Lats	Upper and lower back
Shrug	3 sets × 8 reps	Trapezius	
Straight-leg dead-lift	3 sets × 8 reps	Erector spinae	
Sit-up (crunches)	3 sets × 15 reps	Rectus abdominus	Abdominals and Trunk
Sit-ups (piked)	3 sets × 15 reps		
Side bends	3 sets × 15 reps	External obliques	

Schedules A and B should each be undertaken three times per week on alternate days.

Weight can easily be raised by increasing body fat content but this is hardly ever desirable. Except in exceptional activities like long-distance swimming and Japanese Somo wrestling the really successful sportsman seldom has a great deal of fat. Even Olympic shot-putters, who might be expected to benefit from the extra weight, seem to have no more fat than the average man (Tanner 1964). The top level power-eventer has a great deal of muscle and it tends to be the less successful competitors who accumulate fat.

Body-building is a sport in its own right with a wide following. The majority of body-builders seem to develop muscle by relatively few repetitions of very heavy lifts and later attempt to improve muscle definition with rapid repetitions with light weights. It is common to use 30–40 repetitions per set. Dietary supplements of protein, vitamins, minerals and other substances are widely advertised in body-building magazines. While an adequate intake of these substances is necessary there is no good evidence that excessive quantities help muscular development. In the only carefully controlled study on the use of protein supplements in body-building that is known to the author, the results were negative (Rasch *et al.* 1969).

DECREASING BODY WEIGHT

Body weight can be reduced through a loss of either water or fat. The former leads to dehydration which degrades athletic performance and is particularly undesirable in endurance events, being likely to result in early heat stroke. The weight loss which follows a period of intensive exercise can usually be attributed to water loss and is quickly reversed. Boxers and wrestlers often lose a considerable amount of water in the process of 'making weight'. Some of this is replaced between the weigh-in and the fight.

It is very difficult to give specific advice on reducing fat content because of variations in the distribution of fat deposits between individuals and because of the strong influence of genetic factors on body fat content (Mayer 1953; Sheilds 1962; Osbourne and De George 1959; Brooke *et al.* 1975). In a three-year study of young sportsmen it was found that the fat content of individuals low in endomorphy remained approximately constant irrespective of the state of nutrition and training, while in other subjects quite wide fluctuations occurred (Watson 1979). Individuals high in endomorphy tend to accumulate fat with increasing age. Young endomorphs may not have a great deal of fat but due to the likelihood of increases occurring in the future they should be steered away from activities where fatness is a particular handicap.

Fat reduction may be approached in two ways: through exercise and by manipulation of the diet. Excessive calories cause fat to accumulate, and foods vary widely in their calorific content. Carbohydrate and protein contain only 44 per cent of the calories of an equal weight of fat. In addition, many protein and carbohydrate based foods contain large amounts of water which is inert. For example, potatoes contain 80 per

Fig. 4.18 Superficial
muscles of the abdomen
and thorax.

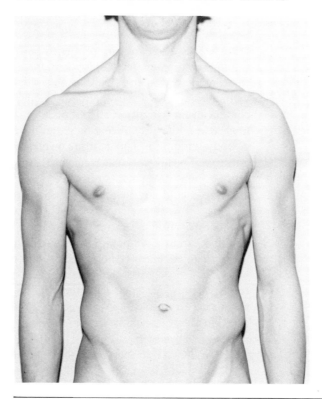

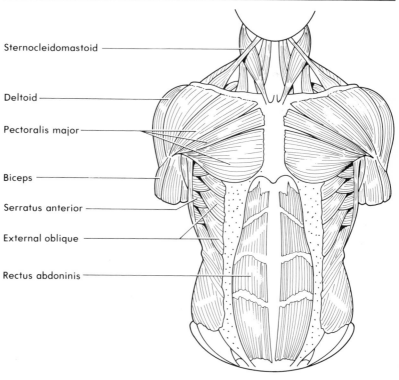

Sternocleidomastoid

Deltoid

Pectoralis major

Biceps

Serratus anterior

External oblique

Rectus abdoninis

cent water and only about 19 per cent carbohydrate. Thus a pound of potatoes contains only 9 per cent of the calories of an equal weight of butter. Thus the elimination of fried and fatty foods from the diet and the substitution of fish or chicken for animal meat will help reduce calorific intake. Sugary snacks should also be avoided.

Increasing the level of physical activity leads to a reduction in fat content in most, but not all, individuals. Since fat deposits are used by muscle as a fuel only during light and moderate exercise, longer periods of work at one-third to half the maximum rate ought to be the most effective. During very vigorous work glycogen is used as fuel and most of the weight loss consists of sweat. Two recent studies suggest that exercise in a cold environment is particularly favourable for fat loss, especially if food intake is restricted (O'Hara *et al.* 1977, 1979).

Some sportsmen are troubled by exccessive deposits of fat in a particular location – commonly the legs, thighs, abdomen or buttocks. In addition to increasing body weight this may reduce anaerobic power output. Such deposits may be extremely difficult to reduce and no systematic study of 'spot reduction' in young athletes is known. The author has experimented with various approaches: rapid full-range exercises involving the body part in question against negligible resistance, jogging in airtight plastic pants, weight training exercises. All have resulted in favourable changes in some individuals.

PLYOMETRICS – BOUNDING EXERCISES

These are most frequently used as a means of increasing speed and anaerobic power output in sprinters and jumpers, but the technique may also be of value to other types of sportsmen. In an unpublished study, Hennessy (1981) found that the programme described below produced favourable results when compared with the effects of two different types of weight training.

Before beginning a programme of bounding the athlete needs a reasonable level of all-round fitness and should be used to jumping, sprinting and stretching. Good training shoes with well padded soles and heels are necessary. A thorough warm-up is essential. This might consist of jogging ¼–½ mile followed by stretching exercises with particular emphasis being paid to the quads, hamstrings, calves, back and hip flexion. The five bounding exercises described below are illustrated in Fig. 4.19.

1. Leap frog. The objective is to propel the body into the air from the full-squat position. The athlete moves upwards and forwards and endeavours to cover as much ground as possible.

2. Hopping. A single-leg hop in which the athlete attempts to gain height as well as distance. The take-off leg undertakes a pumping action, being fully extended on landing.

3. Bounding strides. The athlete endeavours to travel as far as possible trying to obtain height as well as distance.

Fig. 4.19 Bounding exercises. (Courtesy Liam Hennessy.)

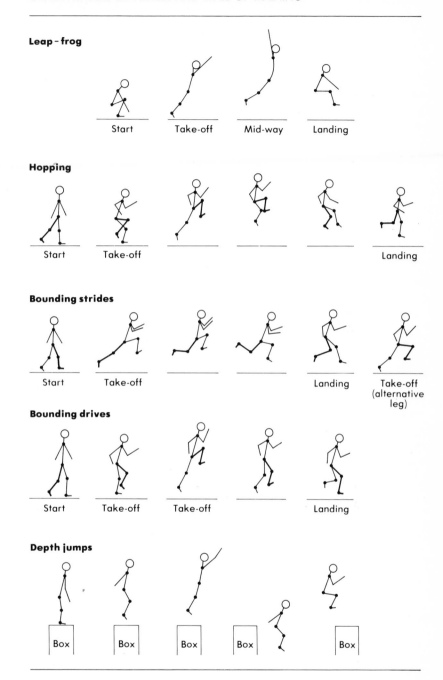

Leap-frog

Start Take-off Mid-way Landing

Hopping

Start Take-off Landing

Bounding strides

Start Take-off Landing Take-off (alternative leg)

Bounding drives

Start Take-off Take-off Landing

Depth jumps

Box Box Box Box Box

4. Bounding drives. Similar to the exercise above except that the athlete attempts to gain height only. A straight take-off is used. Note the straight body position and full extension of the hip in the middle phase of the exercise.

131

5. Depth jumps. The athlete starts the exercise standing on a box and takes off upwards and forwards. He lands on the floor bending his knees and landing on the balls of his feet, then immediately propels himself upwards and forwards onto a second box. Ten such jumps should be used per set. Begin with a box height of 0.5 metre or less and progress up to a maximum of 1.5 metres.

During the first two to three sessions the athlete learns the exercises. During the following week he performs one set of 10 repetitions of each exercise at each session. One further set of each exercise is added each week so that by the fifth week five sets of 10 repetitions of each exercise are being performed. The athlete should train three times per week, if possible on alternate days.

Plyometrics may be adapted for upper body work by the use of some heavy object like a medicine ball.

GENERAL METHODS OF TRAINING

CALLISTHENICS

This term means different things to different people but such training frequently consists of a series of exercises designed to improve flexibility or strength, or both. Such a programme may contain flexibility exercises combined with work against body weight resistance, such as push-ups or sit-ups. Callisthenics are unlikely to produce such large increases in fitness as the more specialised programmes previously discussed, but for many non-athletes this is unlikely to matter. Significant gains in strength, flexibility, and even endurance, are possible if the initial levels are low.

CIRCUIT TRAINING

This method of training consists of a series of exercises done in rotation. When one set of each has been completed the series is performed again, three sets being usual. It is possible to construct circuits which emphasise different aspects of fitness – strength, muscular endurance, speed, flexibility or even skill. The most common type stresses strength and local anaerobic endurance. It is usual to perform the exercise successively and against the clock. This will overload the cardiovascular system and result in an increase in aerobic capacity if the initial level is low. Circuit training is thus a way of developing all-round fitness. As with callisthenics, it is unlikely that any particular aspect will respond as positively as to other specialised forms of training, but useful gains are possible and the method is often employed by sports teams. Circuit training is extremely adaptable and with efficient organisation larger numbers of individuals can be accommodated with the minimum of time, space and equipment. Many different variations are given by Morgan and Adamson (1961) and Sorani (1966). The organisation of one type of circuit is summarised below:

1. Suitable exercises are selected. Usually between 6 and 12 in number.

2. The subjects are taught to perform these **correctly**.

3. Each subject determines the maximum number of repetitions per minute for each exercise (or the maximum number if this is less).

4. The scores are **halved** and recorded on a card which the subject retains. These are the repetitions that the subject will perform in each circuit.

5. At the first training session the subject completes three circuits, each consisting of one set of each exercise. This is done as quickly as possible and the time is recorded. It should be emphasised that the exercises must be performed correctly using the full range of movement.

6. At subsequent sessions individuals attempt to improve on their time.

7. When the time has been reduced by 20 per cent the individual's maximum for each exercise is reassessed and steps 4 to 6 repeated. An alternative way of determining the training dosage is to find the maximum number of repetitions possible in 30 seconds and to use half to three-quarters of this value in each circuit.

Exercises which may be used in a programme of circuit training include:

1. *Using no equipment.* Running on the spot, 10 metre sprints, shuttle runs, squat jumps, leg lifts, press-ups (push-ups), lateral leg raisers, double lateral leg raisers, squat thrusts, hip raisers, back shuffle (similar to squat thrusts but performed supine), sit-ups, V-sits.

2. *With equipment.* Bench stepping (one foot at a time), bench astride jumps, bench astride jumps with weights, rope climb, chins, dips, sit-ups on an incline, press-ups with the feet raised, knee extensions, back extensions, leg extensions, travelling along parallel bars on the hands, travelling along a raised ladder with the hands, rope-ladder climb, squat-and-press with bench.

3. *With weights.* Sideways dumb-bell raising, barbell press, barbell swings, barbell curls, barbell squats, bench press, straight-leg dead-lift, triceps extension, bent-arm pull-over, straight-arm pull-over, supine side dumb-bell raise, wrist rolling. Some of these exercises are illustrated in Fig. 4.20.

It is helpful to prepare posters describing each exercise; these can be fixed to the wall at the site of the activity. One variation of circuit training that is useful for large groups consists of allowing a fixed time of 30 seconds or 1 minute for each activity. This is marked by the blowing of a whistle. The subject performs as many repetitions as he can in this time and records his progress as the increase in the number of repetitions.

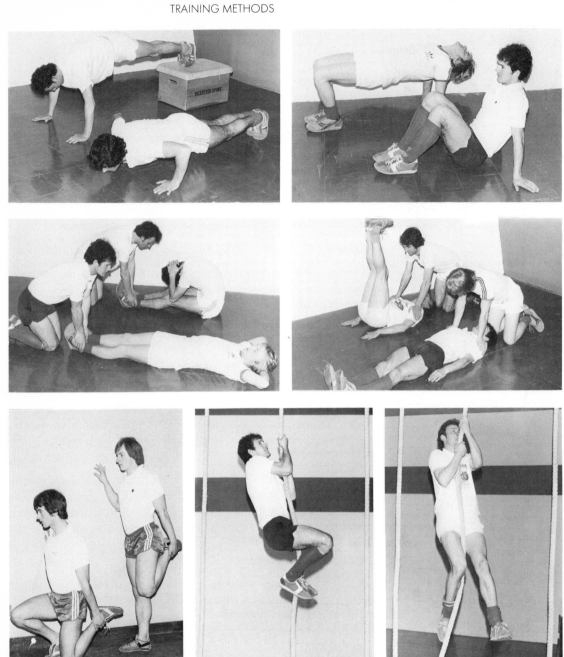

Fig. 4.20 Circuit training
exercises.

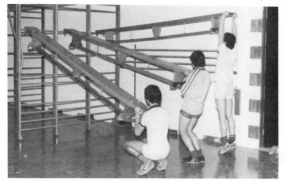

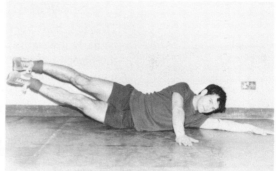

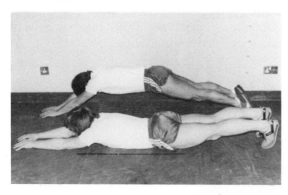

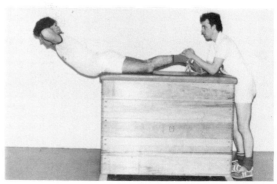

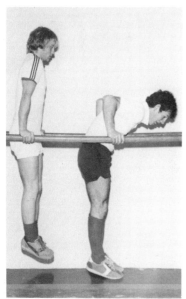

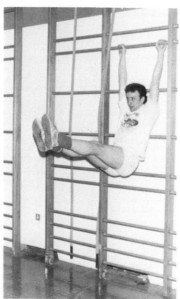

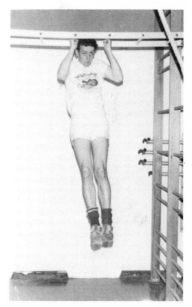

CIRCUIT WEIGHT TRAINING

This is a convenient way of accommodating a group of subjects, particularly if weight-training machines are available. Standard lifts such as the biceps curl, bench press and leg press are used. A typical arrangement is to have each subject undertake 8–10 different exercises in each of two or three circuits. Between 10 and 20 repetitions of half the 1 R.M. are used and the subject is allowed to rest for 20–30 seconds after each exercise. A typical circuit weight-training programme might include the following exercises: bench press, inclined sit-up, leg press, lats pull, back arch, shoulder press, leg extension, arm curl, leg flexion, upright row.

Circuit weight training increases strength and there may also be changes in anaerobic endurance (Wilmore *et al*. 1978). Improvements in aerobic capacity are small, if they occur at all (Gettman *et al*. 1978).

5 EVALUATION OF FITNESS LEVELS

Previous sections have stressed the need to construct training programmes around the demands of particular sports activities. It is equally necessary to take into account the training needs of the individual. Table 5.1 gives fitness profiles of three boxers who were preparing for the 1980 Olympics.

A. J. was already highly successful, being a Commonwealth Games gold medallist. F. L. was a national champion and B. C. a junior champion, a newcomer to the senior squad. A. J.'s success is reflected in his fitness scores which, with the exception of that for endurance, are all above the 80th percentile. In contrast F. L. had a high score for endurance but was low in muscular strength. The younger boxer lacked both strength and endurance. The strength measurements substantiated the observations made by the team coaches and also helped to pin-point particular areas of weakness. As a result of these tests it was possible to devise training programmes that suited each boxer's needs.

Two different approaches to evaluation are illustrated in the paragraph above. Subjective assessment made through observation of the athlete during actual competition, and objective assessment using laboratory techniques. Both methods are capable of providing potentially useful information; both have certain drawbacks.

Table 5.1 Fitness profiles of three boxers

	Boxer		
	A.J.	F.L.	B.C.
Endurance (aerobic)	65	92	29
Flexibility	97	24	36
Strength: arm	95	17	32
back	83	50	56
Speed	85	78	40
Fat (%)	13	8	15
Posture	OK	OK	Lordosis

Scores for endurance, flexibility, strength and speed are percentiles (100 = maximum score), adjusted for differences in body weight.

SUBJECTIVE EVALUATION

With subjective evaluation it is not easy to distinguish fitness from performance, or to isolate one component of fitness from another. A champion pole-vaulter is, almost by definition, very fit for that particular activity. But it may be difficult to know whether his success is due to vaulting technique, sprinting speed, leg or upper-body strength. If he wishes to improve his performance further it is important to know which of these should be developed. Figure 5.1 shows the result of a comparison of various subjective assessments of aerobic endurance with a laboratory measurement. They were made by a lecturer in physical education who was running a conditioning course, three students who had experience as team trainers, and three laymen. Before the investigation it was anticipated that the lecturer's assessment would be most highly related to the laboratory measure, and that the students' efforts would be useful but less accurate.

In fact only the assessment made by student B had a significant positive relationship to endurance. The assessment of one of the laymen had a significant negative relationship to the laboratory measure. When the participants were asked how they arrived at their scores it was clear that student B was influenced by his knowledge of the subject's training

Fig. 5.1 Correlation and percentage of common variance between an objective measure of aerobic endurance and subjective estimates made by seven individuals. (Data from Watson 1978.)

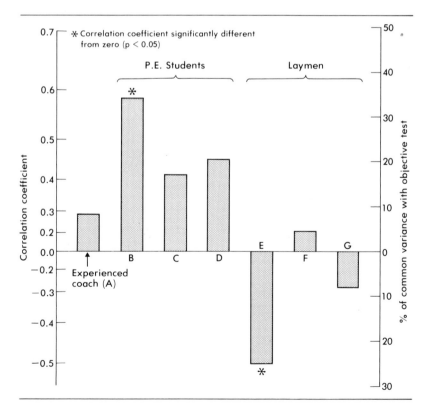

habits. Layman F had difficulty in identifying aerobic endurance and his assessment was influenced by the subject's physique. This study illustrates how difficult it is to assess fitness subjectively even when the observer is very experienced. The efforts of student B and layman F are probably typical of many subjective evaluations, being influenced by variables other than those that were actually being examined.

Subjective assessment is capable of providing useful information in certain circumstances. The subject should be observed in a situation where the variable in question can be easily identified and in circumstances where it can be clearly differentiated from other factors. During a game or a training session it is not always easy to isolate endurance from skill and experience, because a more skilful individual may perform with greater efficiency and achieve the same results with a lower energy expenditure.

If the subjective evaluation of fitness is to be successful it is necessary to identify the relevant variables and to establish a procedure for isolating each one from other factors. With many aspects of fitness it is necessary to distinguish between subcomponents. For example, strength must be subdivided into static and dynamic forms and particular muscle groups should be considered. Lastly, the criteria for the evaluation of each item need to be established. It is unlikely that a useful assessment will result unless all this is done.

When undertaken systematically, subjective evaluation can provide valuable information. Its strength is the relevance to particular sporting activities. It has been shown earlier that components of fitness are high-

Fig. 5.2 An approach to the subjective evaluation of physical fitness variables.

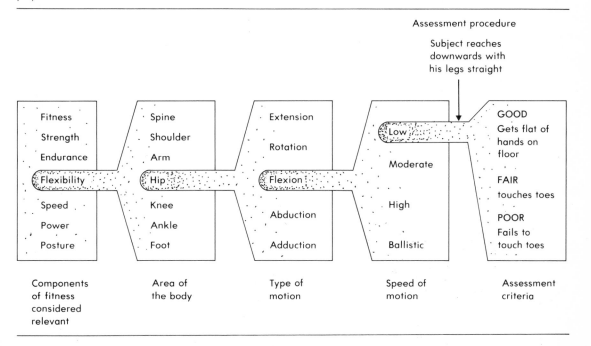

ly specific. Many laboratory procedures measure aspects of performance that are not precisely duplicated during athletic competition and this makes their interpretation difficult. Short of producing a different instrument for every sporting situation, it is simply not possible to take all the measurements necessary for the quantification of fitness as it is expressed in different activities. The gap must be filled by subjective evaluation. It is a very large gap indeed. Subjective evaluation also has its limitations. The difficulty of differentiating the various components of fitness has already been mentioned. Even if this problem is successfully overcome the information obtained may be of limited diagnostic value. Subjective evaluation is often too general to pin-point a particular problem. It is also difficult to make consistent observations and to eliminate bias. A measurement that appears on a dial is perfectly neutral and the instrument that produces it takes no account of the personality or history of the subject. When making a subjective assessment it is very difficult to forget that X has missed the last four training sessions and that his sense of humour makes you cringe. Even if you do forget, the information may still have a subconscious impact.

QUANTITATIVE METHODS OF ASSESSING FITNESS

In this section the term 'quantitative' is used where a measurement occurs on a continuous numerical scale and does not result from the judgement of the observer. In these terms 'height' and 'weight' are quantitative measurements but the scores of a judge at a diving competition are not.

Quantitative measurements avoid some of the disadvantages of subjective assessment. They are not influenced by personal interactions and are usually less subject to error.

In order to be useful a measuring procedure must satisfy two basic demands. It must tell us something we want to know and it must do so consistently, so that a repeat measurement will be closely similar to the original. The first requirement is simply a matter of selecting the right test and would not appear difficult to satisfy. But suppose we want to know the percentage of fat in an athlete's body. The only accurate method of measuring this involves removing all the fat and weighing it. This is obviously not practicable and it is necessary to find another way that leaves the subject intact. There are several methods available which allow fat content to be *estimated*. They give results that approximate to the direct measurement. The amount of agreement is sometimes known as the **validity** of the estimate. For a test to be useful it must normally have a high validity, but convenience and the purpose of the test must also be taken into account. A rough estimate of endurance is probably all that is needed in the case of a housewife who wants to take up jogging. It would be a waste of time and effort to go to the trouble of making a direct measurement of $\dot{V}_{O, max}$, or even of obtaining an accurate estimate. On the other hand, if a new training technique is being evaluated a test with high validity is essential.

A test must also give results that are reproducible. This is important because differences in score will usually be interpreted as changes in fitness. If the test is unreliable such changes may simply be due to errors of measurement. Figure 5.3 illustrates a typical study of the reliability of a fitness test. PWC_{170} was measured on two occasions, separated by 24 hours, in a group of 29 individuals; 19 were students who had undertaken the test before and the other 9 were schoolboys who were new to the test. The percentage change in score when the measurement was repeated is shown for each subject. If the results for the students are considered it can be seen that in most cases there were slight variations in score between the two attempts. The differences range from a gain of 7.5 per cent to a loss of 6.5 per cent. The average is 0 per cent and this indicates that these are random errors. They are due to chance variations in the measuring instruments, or the way they were read by the observer, or the physiology of the subjects. Upon investigation the errors in this particular test were attributed primarily to the last cause. The standard deviation of the changes is ± 3 per cent. Statistical tables indicate that 95 per cent of all scores would be expected to lie within ±2 standard deviations of the mean. In this case 95

Fig. 5.3 Changes in PWC_{170} score when 19 experienced and 10 novice subjects were tested then re-tested 24 hours later. (From Watson and O'Donovan 1976 b).

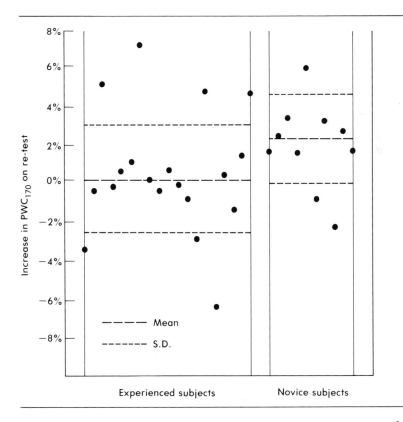

per cent of repeat measurements would be expected to be accurate to within ±6 per cent. This is the reliability of this test as conducted in one particular set of circumstances. If the equipment had been in a poorer condition, or if the observer had been less skilled or less careful, the error would have been greater. In this case we can be 95 per cent certain that a subject who obtains a score of 1,000 units has an actual value somewhere between 940 and 1,060. If he took the test again after a month and obtained a score of 1,020 it would not be justifiable to conclude that he had increased his fitness.

Reliability is often expressed in terms of the test–re-test correlation. In the example above this happened to be 0.98. The method is less satisfactory than the procedure described above because it is more difficult to interpret and because the correlation coefficient is influenced by the spread of scores as well as their scatter. An example is given in Fig. 5.7. Each individual's re-test score is plotted on the Y (or vertical) axis against his test score on the X (or horizontal) axis. In Fig. 5.7 the 95 per cent confidence limits of reproducibility are ±7 per cent despite the test–re-test correlation being only 0.6999.

The right-hand portion of Fig. 5.3 shows the change in score of the schoolboys. The random variations are similar to those for the students but in this case there is also a systematic error, because the mean change in score is greater than zero. Systematic errors move all scores in the same direction. They are due to a variety of causes including changes in the subjects, the equipment, or the administration of the test. One of the most common sources of systematic error is gradual changes in measuring equipment such as stop-watches running slow, tape measures stretching and the springs in weighing machines and dynamometers becoming slack. Changes in the opposite direction are also possible.

It is important to calibrate all instruments on a regular basis and to standardise the measuring techniques very rigorously. In the author's experience systematic errors usually cause more serious problems than the random variety. Teachers and students usually measure consistently within one particular session, but long-term studies are hampered by changes in technique or instrument calibration. Listed below are some points which will help to increase reliability:

1. Calibrate all instruments before each session of measurement.
2. Standardise the measuring technique.
3. Record all observations immediately.
4. Standardise the testing location, and the kit and footwear of the subjects.
5. Try to take repeat measurements at the same time of day.
6. Try to standardise the temperature and humidity of the testing environment.
7. Do not conduct tests on subjects who have just eaten or taken any form of exercise.

8. Follow a consistent organisational procedure in terms of the number and type of subjects tested at one time, otherwise the level of motivation may vary.

9. Standardise the amount of warm-up and practice allowed.

10. Record all details of the test protocol and the measuring techniques employed.

SPECIFIC TYPES OF MEASUREMENTS

STRENGTH

Isometric strength

Aspects of isometric strength may be measured using the dynamometers illustrated in Fig. 5.4. These instruments give stable readings and are exceptionally easy to use. Calibration can be carried out using a set of known weights. The 95 per cent confidence limits of reproducibility are typically within ±8 per cent.

The cable tensiometer (illustrated in Fig. 5.5) is a universal dynamometer which can be adapted to measure the strength of most muscle groups. It is a versatile instrument but is considerably more troublesome to use than the simple dynamometers illustrated in Fig. 5.4.

Isometric strength is a reasonable indicator of dynamic strength in sedentary individuals but is less likely to be a good guide in those who have trained using other types of muscle contraction. The author is aware of throwers with only moderate scores in isometric strength despite high levels of isokinetic strength and the ability to lift heavy weights. In sportsmen tests of isometric strength are most useful for the assessment of muscle groups which act in a stabilising capacity during physical activity.

Notes on the use of strength-measuring dynamometers

1. The results of all strength tests may be influenced by the level of motivation. The subjects should be encouraged to produce maximum effort. It is often easier to achieve this if a group of individuals work in competition.

2. The correct procedure for each test should be demonstrated to the subject and he should then be allowed two or three attempts. These should be separated from each other by a rest period of at least 2 minutes.

3. When measuring hand grip the dynamometer grip size should be adjusted to suit the size of the subject's hand. The dynamometer should be gripped near the end of the fingers otherwise it may slip inwards when pressure is apppplied.

4. With all dynamometer tests, sweat should be removed from the in-

Fig. 5.4 Measurement of isometric strength: (a) hand-grip; (b) push and pull; (c) leg; (d) back.

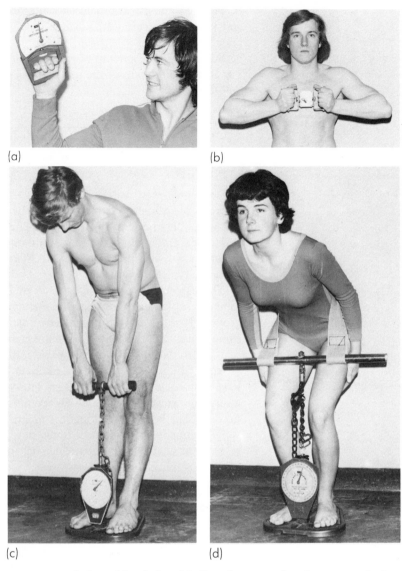

(a)　　　　　　(b)

(c)　　　　　　(d)

strument and the subject's hand before the start of each attempt. In hot weather French chalk should be applied to both.

5. With the back- and leg-strength tests the dynamometer chain length should be adjusted to suit the subject's height. In the author's experience the precise length of the chain is not as important as is sometimes suggested, but it is advisable to maintain a constant length for repeat tests on one subject.

6. With the push and pull tests the subject's arms and the dynamometer should be held in a straight line.

7. In the back-strength test the subject must not be allowed to supple-

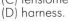

Fig. 5.5 The cable tensiometer. (A) Secure hook in wall; (B) cable; (C) tensiometer; (D) harness.

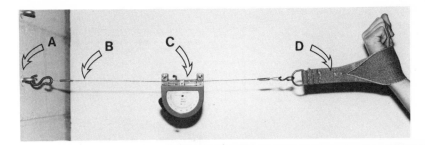

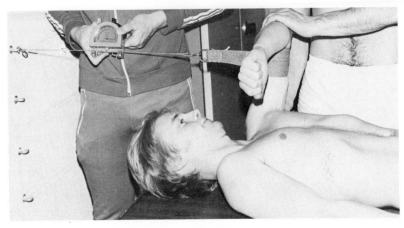

ment his score by the use of the legs. The tester must ensure that the subject's knees are fully hyper-extended throughout the measurement.

8. When using the cable tensiometer it is important that the subject is adequately supported so that force is exerted only by the muscle group being tested. As with other isometric strength tests it is necessary to standardise the joint angle at which each measurement is taken.

Dynamic strength
Strength increases brought about through weight training are indicated by the rising repetition maximum (R.M.). As illustrated in Fig. 4.6 (p. 98), the increase may be specific to the type of training employed and will not necessarily reflect the gains in strength when a different type of contraction is used.

Measurement of strength without the use of instruments
Many test batteries use the maximum number of repetitions of a particular movement as an indicator of strength. Such exercises as leg lifts, sit-ups, push-ups, dips, chins, squat thrusts and squat jumps are examples. Strictly, these are measures of muscular endurance rather than strength but the two are closely related and such tests can give a reasonable indication of strength. Many of these exercises are influenced by body weight but since the ability of the individual to propel himself is subject to similar constraints, this is often not a serious disadvantage.

Fig. 5.6 Battery of cable tensiometer tests.

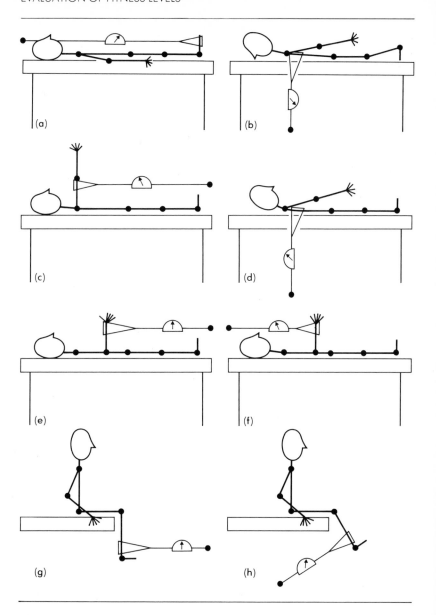

Such tests can provide useful information when no measuring instruments are available. It is not important how each exercise is performed as long as the method is standardised between the individuals tested and between attempts. New exercises can be devised to test particular muscle groups. The results are most likely to approximate to strength scores when the number of repetitions is reasonably low. If this is not the case, the exercise should be made more difficult. For example, sit-ups can be performed on an incline or with the subject holding a weight behind his head.

Fig. 5.7 Reliability of the Margaria power test. Re-test scores are plotted on the vertical axis against test scores on the horizontal axis. The test–re-test correlation is only 0.699 but this is partly due to the small range of scores. The reliability of the test is to within ± 7 per cent.

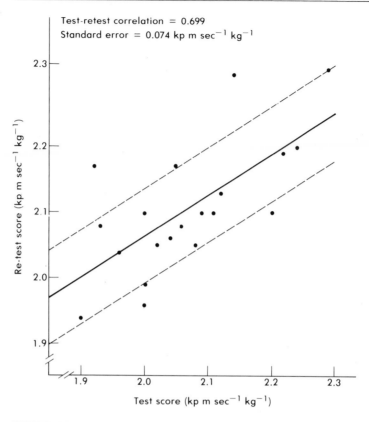

ANAEROBIC POWER OUTPUT (ALACTIC)

The measurement of this important aspect of fitness has not received the attention it deserves. The best established test is that described by Margaria and his colleagues (1966). The subject runs up a flight of about 12 steps. Photo-cells or switch mats are placed on the third and ninth steps and the subject is timed through a vertical distance of about 1 metre. The test seems to work best if the run-up to the steps is confined to a horizontal distance of 2–3 metres.

A certain amount of skill is required to bound up a flight of steps two or three at a time, and this causes difficulties in some subjects. On the other hand, highly coordinated individuals are able to devise a strategy for 'cheating' the timing device and this can inflate their scores by up to 10 per cent. In a study carried out on a cross-section of sportsmen the author found that the reliability of the test was optimised if each subject was allowed 10 attempts at the test and power output was then computed from the mean of the best five attempts. The reliability of the Margaria test, as carried out under these conditions, is illustrated in Fig. 5.7.

147

Power output can be calculated either as raw power:

$$\text{power} = \frac{\text{body weight} \times \text{vertical distance between timing devices}}{\text{time}}$$

or as power per kg body weight:

$$\frac{\text{power}}{\text{per kg}} = \frac{\cancel{\text{body weight}} \times \text{vertical distance between timing devices}}{\text{time} \times \cancel{\text{body weight}}}$$

$$= \frac{\text{vertical distance between timing devices}}{\text{time}}$$

Example: distance between timing devices   1.06 m
time   0.469 s
body weight of subject   65.00 kg

$$\text{power output} = \frac{65.00 \times 1.06}{0.469} = 146.9 \text{ kp m s}^{-1}$$

$$\frac{\text{power per kg}}{\text{of body weight}} = \frac{1.06}{0.469} = 2.26 \text{ kp m s}^{-1} \text{ kg}^{-1}$$

In the study quoted above it was found that 70 per cent of the variance in raw power scores was accounted for by differences in body weight and only 30 per cent by variations in run time. Thus, the second equation is generally the most satisfactory method of comparing the power output of different individuals.

Other methods of estimating alactic power output are: (1) using the vertical jump test and (2) from the time for a 50 yard dash. In the latter a 15 yard running start is used and the subjects are compared on the basis of their speed.

Alactic power output can be estimated from vertical jump scores by means of the following equation:

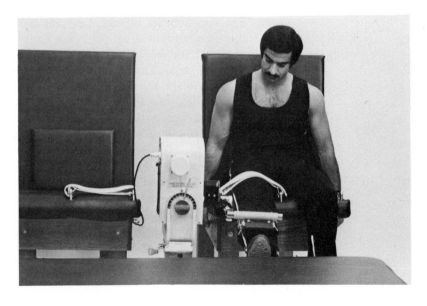

Fig. 5.8 An isokinetic dynamometer. This device measures the force that can be produced at constant speed of movement. (Courtesy Lumex Inc., New York.)

power output = $2.2 \times$ body weight $\times \sqrt{\mathcal{J}}$
(kp m s^{-1})   (kg)

where $\mathcal{J}$ is the height jumped in metres. $\mathcal{J}$ is measured as the difference between the subject's standing reach and his reach at the height of the jump.

The above three tests measure power output during work that is done primarily with the legs. The alactic power output of other muscle groups can be assessed using isokinetic dynamometers. These are now commercially available although expensive. An example is illustrated in Fig. 5.8.

Alactic power is vital in any explosive event but is specific to the speed of motion as well as to the muscle groups involved. There is a need to develop ways of measuring the power output achieved in particular activities. This would enable training methods to be improved.

ENDURANCE

1. Alactic endurance
This can be measured as the power output achieved during an activity that lasts for a few seconds. Many of the procedures described for the assessment of power can be modified to provide a measure of alactic endurance. An upstairs run lasting 5–10 seconds is an example. In such tests performance is determined by the availability of anaerobic energy sources to muscle, rather than by neuro-muscular coordination.

2. Lactic endurance
It is impossible to measure this variable directly because of the complex nature of lactic acid metabolism. The maximum concentration of lactic acid in muscle or blood is some guide but, as discussed in Chapter 2, such scores are difficult to interpret.

A number of authors have described tests in which the subject works on a treadmill or bicycle ergometer at a rate in excess of his aerobic capacity. The maximum duration of such exercise is taken as a measure of lactic endurance. A useful example is based on work by Cunningham and Faulkner (1969) as used by Houston and Thomson (1977). The subject runs on a treadmill set to a speed of 215 metres per minute and a slope of 20 per cent. Scores normally range between 30 and 100 seconds. When carrying out this test on novice subjects it is important to allow some practice at running on the treadmill. Motivation is an important factor and scores tend to improve after the initial attempt. At least two attempts are necessary if the results are to be reliable.

Aerobic endurance
This is also known as *aerobic capacity* and *physical working capacity* (PWC).

It can be determined in a number of ways, including measurement of the maximum consumption of oxygen and the work that can be done at a given submaximal heart rate. Endurance tests are also used as a measure of aerobic capacity.

This area of measurement has received more attention than any other and the variety of different procedures is wide. The features of some of the more useful and important tests are considered below.

Maximum oxygen uptake   The principle of this method is considered but no detailed description given since this is a technique that can be acquired only through experience in a laboratory. In essence the procedure is quite straightforward. The subject exercises at a gradually increasing rate while his oxygen consumption is monitored. Any mode of exercise can be used but a treadmill or bicycle ergometer is most commonly employed. The subject's oxygen consumption increases with his rate of working and gradually reaches a peak as illustrated in Fig. 5.9. The maximum value is recorded as an indication of the subject's capacity for aerobic work.

It is usually possible to increase the work load even after the maximum uptake of oxygen has been achieved. This extra work is done anaerobically. Maximum oxygen uptake is thus a measure of the capacity for aerobic rather than total work. In theory, $\dot{V}_{O_2\text{max}}$ should reach a plateau and then remain steady. In practice there are usually fluctuations and it is then necessary to make an arbitrary decision as to the maximum value. Several different criteria for establishing this have

Fig. 5.9 Oxygen intake at increasing work-loads. The value eventually reaches a maximum which is known as the 'maximum oxygen uptake' or $\dot{V}_{O_2\text{max}}$.

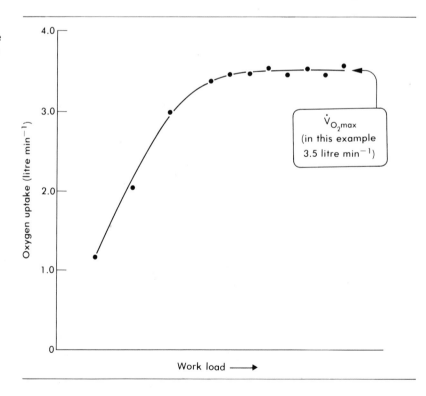

been proposed by different workers (e.g. Taylor *et al.* 1955; Mitchell *et al.* 1958; Balke and Ware 1959). Glassford *et al.* (1965) found only 50 per cent of common variance between three standard methods of measuring $\dot{V}_{O_2\,max}$ and Froelicher *et al.* (1974) report systematic differences of 9.7 per cent.

In measuring maximum oxygen uptake the greatest difficulty lies in the collection and estimation of gases. It is usual to collect the air that the subject has expired and analyse it for oxygen content. During maximum exercise the oxygen extracted amounts to only 2–5 per cent of the total volume of air. This means that the effect of any error in oxy-

Fig. 5.10 Determination of maximum oxygen uptake: (*top*) during running on a treadmill; (*bottom*) during simulated kyaking. (Photograph by kind permission of Dr F.S. Pike.)

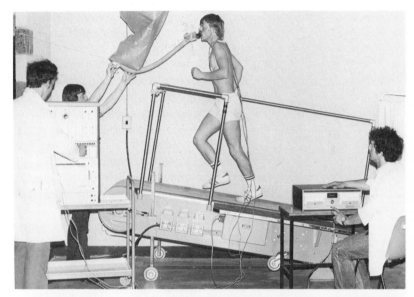

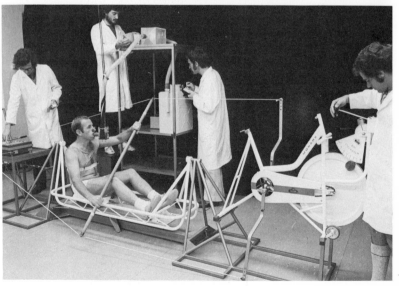

gen analysis is multiplied 20–50 times when oxygen uptake is computed. Very precise methods of gas analysis are required and frequent calibration of instruments is essential. The collection of gases also presents difficulties. It is not easy to avoid leaks and the design and construction of mouthpieces and valve units can have an important influence on the measured uptake of the subject. Under ideal conditions the reliability of the maximum oxygen uptake test is probably about ±6 per cent. But it is unlikely that this is often achieved and there are probably much greater systematic errors between measurements made in different laboratories. In an attempt to investigate systematic errors in oxygen analysis Cotes and Woolmer (1962) had a cylinder of gas tested for oxygen content in six different laboratories that specialised in this type of work. The differences would have resulted in variations in $\dot{V}_{O_2 \, max}$ of up to 25 per cent. Bonjer (1966) found similar discrepancies in analyses by Dutch laboratories. When the effects of differences in gas collection equipment and experimental procedure are added to these errors of gas analysis the variations in $\dot{V}_{O_2 \, max}$ may be very large indeed.

It is necessary to be very cautious about measurements of maximum oxygen uptake unless they have an impeccable pedigree. The quantity *can* be determined with accuracy but first-class equipment and experienced personnel are required. If either of these ingredients is missing it may be better to estimate aerobic capacity by other methods. Coaches need to be cautious of determinations of $\dot{V}_{O_2 \, max}$ determination made by inexperienced individuals.

There may also be difficulties of interpretation. For many years aerobic capacity was assumed to be a central phenomenon, determined solely by the efficiency of the cardio-respiratory system. It is now known that muscle biochemistry also has an important influence. A subject's $\dot{V}_{O_2 \, max}$ may be highest when particular muscle groups are used. Improvements in $\dot{V}_{O_2 \, max}$ due to training are often apparent only when the subject is tested using the mode of exercise employed during training (see Chs 2, 3 and 4). These findings indicate that $\dot{V}_{O_2 \, max}$ is not the unambiguous indicator of the capacity for aerobic work that is often suggested. The standard treadmill $\dot{V}_{O_2 \, max}$ test is a useful indicator of the capacity of the cardio-respiratory system. Insofar as this is a component of all endurance-type activities the test does provide useful information about fitness. But it is not a good indicator of improvements in work capacity due to specific types of training unless the test is carried out using the same exercise mode. For example, improvements in the capacity for aerobic work during swimming can be accurately monitored only if maximum oxygen uptake is measured during this type of exercise. There is a need for the development of tests to monitor the effects of specific forms of training.

Estimating maximum oxygen uptake　There are a number of ways of estimating $\dot{V}_{O_2 \, max}$. These involve making a prediction from some other form of measurement and the precision of different estimates varies widely. None is as good as an accurate direct determination of $\dot{V}_{O_2\,max}$, although the best are preferable to an inadequate attempt at this measurement. Estimates are never more reliable than the measuring procedures upon which they are based. Some methods provide a very useful estimate of maximum oxygen uptake but the value of others is questionable. It would be quite easy to produce an equation for the prediction of $\dot{V}_{O_2\,max}$ from resting heart rate – it is probably only a matter of time before someone does. Resting heart-rate is not a good guide to aerobic capacity and any prediction made from it would be no more valuable than the original observation. Some reasonable predictions of $\dot{V}_{O_2\,max}$ can be made from *exercise* heart rates and such methods are considered below.

The original method is due to Astrand and Rhyming (1954). The subject exercises on a bicycle ergometer as described for the PWC_{170} test, except that only one work load is used. This should be selected to produce a final heart rate between 125 and 170 beats per minute. Maximum oxygen uptake is estimated from the nomogram in Fig. 5.11.

A scale is included for the estimation of $\dot{V}_{O_2\,max}$ from step-test pulse rates. The step test is conducted as described below.

The subject steps up and down on a chair or bench, which should be 40 cm high for males and 33 cm for females. The exercise is continued for 6 minutes and 30 steps are made each minute. This involves the subject moving from a standing position on the floor to a standing position on the chair, then back to the floor, 30 times each minute. It is important that he/she stands upright on the chair so that the whole body weight is lifted through the height of the bench. The sequence of steps must be accurately maintained and precautions 3, 4 and 5 of the PWC_{170} test observed.

The subject's pulse is taken for 60 seconds during the final minute of exercise. This is not particularly easy to do unless monitoring equipment is available. In case of difficulty the pulse can be taken during the first 10 seconds of recovery and this value multiplied by 6. Using these methods predictions of $\dot{V}_{O_2\,max}$ are likely to be within ±15 per cent (Davies 1968).

If the Astrand procedure is used with subjects over 25 years of age a correction must be applied to the prediction as shown in Table 5.2

PWC₁₇₀ The PWC_{170} test measures the physical working capacity at a heart rate of 170 beats per minute. That is the amount of work the subject can do when his heart rate is 170 beats per minute. It is a submaximal test of aerobic capacity and is useful because it can be carried out with the minimum of equipment. Figure 5.12 shows what is required.

It is possible to dispense with the stethoscope and measure heart rate from the pulse at the neck. The ergometer is the only major piece of equipment required. The one illustrated is now quite expensive but much cheaper versions are available from suppliers of school science

Fig. 5.11 Nomogram for estimating maximum oxygen uptake from pulse rate during exercise on the bicycle ergometer, or during a step test. The subject's exercise heart rate is joined to the workload (bicycle ergometer test) or to body weight (step test) and the estimate of maximum oxygen uptake read off from the centre scale. In the examples, a female of body weight 61 kg has a heart rate of 156 on the step test; her estimated $\dot{V}_{O_2max}$ is 2.4 litre min^{-1}. A male working with a heart rate of 166 at a work load of 1,200 kp m min^{-1} has an estimated $\dot{V}_{O_2max}$ of 3.6 litre min^{-1} (From Astrand, I. *Acta Physiol. Scand.* 1960, 49 suppl. 169, by kind permission.)

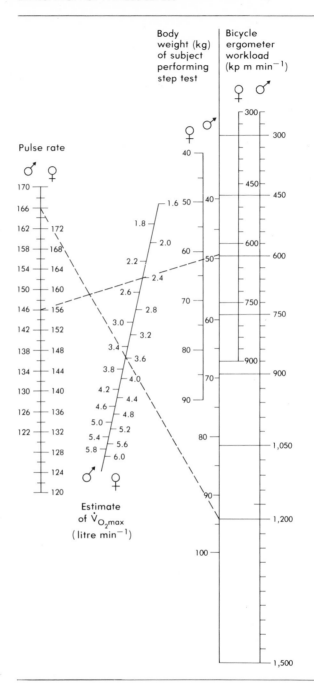

equipment. Any type of ergometer will do as long as it is possible to make an accurate measurement of the work done by the subject.

PWC_{170} scores correlate highly with maximum oxygen uptake. Correlations between 0.86 and 0.91 have been reported by various workers

Table 5.2 Correction factors for subjects over 25 years of age. (For use when making prediction of $\dot{V}_{O_2max}$ from submaximal heart-rates)

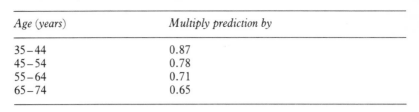

Age (years)	Multiply prediction by
35–44	0.87
45–54	0.78
55–64	0.71
65–74	0.65

Fig. 5.12 Measuring PWC_{170} during a work test on the bicycle ergometer.

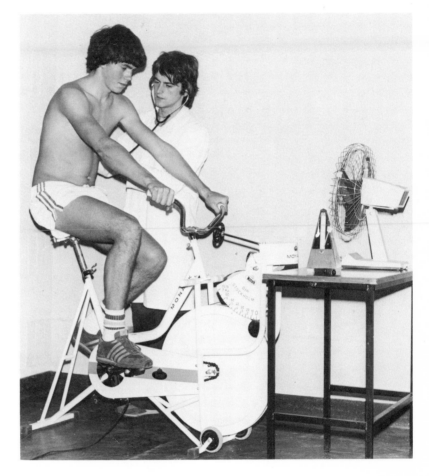

(Cumming and Danziger 1963; Knutten 1967; Watson 1978). The test has been used as a substitute for $\dot{V}_{O_2\ max}$ but is best considered as a separate test because it measures the heart-rate response to submaximal exercise, not maximal aerobic capacity. The two tests give rather different information and both are useful in certain circumstances. $\dot{V}_{O_2\ max}$ is most relevant where the athlete is expected to work flat-out, PWC_{170} for predictions concerning the capacity for submaximal work. Daniels *et al.* (1978a) have found that running ability and PWC_{170} improved with endurance training in a group of pre-puberal boys but that $\dot{V}_{O_2\ max}$ per kg body weight did not change. The present author has also found the

155

PWC_{170} test to be a useful guide to the effects of endurance training in schoolchildren and other young sportsmen.

PWC_{170} is measured by having the subject exercise at two or three different work loads on a bicycle ergometer. The steady state heart rate is measured at each work load and then plotted against the work load as shown in Fig. 5.13. The work load heart-rate plots are then joined by a straight line. PWC_{170} is then obtained as the work load that corresponds to a heart rate of 170 beats per minute.

Several precautions are necessary if an accurate determination is to result:

1. The ergometer must be maintained in good mechanical condition and the force scale zeroed at the start of each measurement.

2. The pedalling rate of the subject and the force setting must be checked once each minute throughout the test.

3. The test should not be carried out following a meal or after a period of exercise.

Fig. 5.13 Computation of PWC_{170}. Where the three points are not exactly aligned the *best* straight line should be drawn.

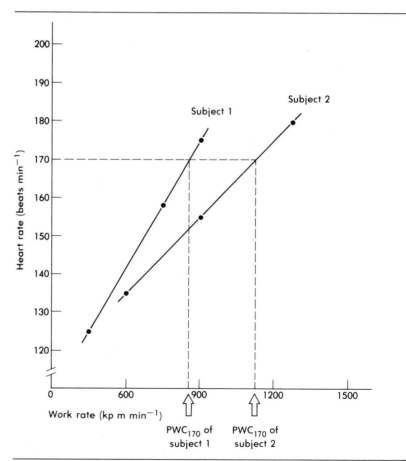

4. The subject should normally work for at least 6 minutes at each work load or until his heart rate becomes steady.

5. The subject should wear a minimum of light clothing and be cooled by a fan. The environment should be cool and the relative humidity low.

6. Steps should be taken to put the subject at ease and to reduce apprehension otherwise the heart rate may be artificially elevated.

Failure to observe precautions 3, 5 and 6 may lead to a low result. Under ideal conditions the PWC_{170} test is reproducible to within ± 6 per cent (see Fig. 5.3). It is possible to shorten the test by reducing the exercise periods to 4 or 5 minutes or by using only two work loads. These modifications do not produce any significant systematic error but reduce the reliability of the test, especially when conducted by an inexperienced observer (Watson and O'Donovan 1976 A).

The 12 minute run-walk test   This is an extremely easy test to administer. The only resources required are a stop-watch and a measured running area. The subjects are instructed to cover as great a distance as they can in 12 minutes by running, walking, or a combination of both. At the end of this period the distance covered is recorded. This is the subject's score.

Several different tests of aerobic capacity have been described in this section. The least complex are the test above and the Astrand step test. Neither requires much equipment and can be carried out in any school or club. Although less precise than the laboratory procedures they are both useful indicators of aerobic fitness.

FLEXIBILITY

Static flexibility is concerned with the range of movement of joints. It can be quantified either as the angle of motion or as the distance through which an extremity of the body travels. Since flexibility measurements are seldom used in mathematical computations it is not usually important which method is used. Angular motion can also be measured from serial X-rays or photographs. In the latter the position of the joint is indicated by markers placed on body prominences.

A device known as a flexiometer can also be used (Leighton 1942). Basically this consists of a dial which is strapped to the limb to be tested, and a pointer which is weighted so that it always remains vertical. The scale moves with the limb so that the angle of motion can be read off from the pointer.

Flexibility is highly specific to individual joints and there is no general test which will give an overall score. It is necessary to measure the range of motion of all joints that are important in a particular situation. This will vary from sport to sport and the coach or trainer is urged to devise tests of his own.

For the reasons stated above it is difficult to select a small number of flexibility tests which are suitable for general use. A battery of simple items which the author has found useful is illustrated in Fig. 5.14. A much wider range of tests of joint function can be obtained from a useful booklet published by the American Academy of Orthopaedic Surgeons (1965).

Battery of static flexibility tests

In the following tests the subject should execute the movement slowly and be required to hold the final position for 5 seconds.

1. *Spinal flexion and hamstring length.* The subject should stand on the box with his feet together. The knees must be fully extended (legs straight) throughout the test. The result is slightly influenced by relative leg length.

2. *Spinal hyper-extension.* The subject stands facing a wall and is supported so that the hips remain in contact with it. The test can also be carried out with the subject lying prone on the floor. It is easier to administer in this form but the result is then influenced by the strength of the subject's back muscles.

3. *Rotation of the spine.* The subject's hips are held in contact with a bench. Movement is measured from flesh marks placed on the centre of each shoulder. Right and left rotation should be measured.

4. *Lateral movement of the spine.* The subject stands with feet hip-width apart. The heels, buttocks, shoulders and head should be in contact with a smooth wall and must remain so throughout the test. With the subject standing upright the position of the tip of the middle finger is marked on the subject's thigh. The subject then leans as far as possible to the left keeping both feet in contact with the floor and the buttocks, shoulders and head in contact with the wall. The vertical distance moved by the tip of the left middle finger is recorded as the subject's score. The test is then repeated on the right-hand side.

5. *Horizontal movement of the arms at the shoulder joint.* The subject should begin the test with arms horizontal. It is important that no vertical movement occurs. Both arms should be moved together.

6. *Hamstring length.* The subject lies supine on a couch or the floor. It is vital that *both* legs remain absolutely straight with the knees fully hyper-extended.

7. *Hip hyper-extension.* The subject's body is supported on a couch. The angle of maximum hyper-extension of one thigh is measured while a helper supports the other leg.

8. *Ankle flexion.* The degree of both dorsi-flexion (x) and plantar flexion (y) should be measured.

9. *Hip abduction.* The subject sits on the floor with his/her heels 6 inches from the groin. The degree of hip abduction is then measured.

In the tests which involve the measurement of lengths (numbers 1, 2 and 4) the results are best expressed as a fraction or percentage of the subject's height. This allows for differences in body size. For example, if a subject of height 1,600 mm obtains a score of +16 mm in test number 1, this is expressed as a fraction of height, a score of 0.01, and a percentage score of 1.000.

ANTHROPOMETRIC MEASUREMENTS

Anthropometric measurements are used to monitor growth and the effects of training. They are also useful as a reference point for the interpretation of other tests since many performance variables are influenced by body size and shape. For this reason measures of strength and aerobic capacity are often expressed per kilogram of body weight.

Height

For very accurate work height is measured using a rigid stadiometer with a massive head-board, but good results can be obtained with just a metre rule and a right-angle wooden triangle. The rule should be fixed to a smooth, vertical wall, 1 metre above the floor. The measurement is then taken by placing the triangle in firm contact with the rule and the top of the subject's head. The subject should stand in bare feet, with his heels together, and in contact with the wall. He should be instructed to stand as 'tall' as possible and to hold his head level so that the face is vertical. This technique will result in measurements that are reproducible to within 5 to 10 mm.

Sitting height

The wooden triangle and metre rule are again used. The subject sits on a table or box of known height with his thighs horizontal and the base of the spine in contact with the metre rule. He should be encouraged to stretch upwards and the measurement is then taken as described for height. The height of the table or box is subtracted from the reading obtained in order to compute sitting height. The measurement is useful as an indication of the length of the trunk. Height minus sitting height is known as *subischial length* and is a reliable measure of leg length. The ratio leg length/trunk length has implications for physical performance. It tends to be high in hurdlers and high jumpers and low in throwers and sprinters.

Weight

Determinations of weight should be made on a reliable set of scales. The bathroom variety can be used for approximate measurements but should be placed on a level surface and adjusted before use. Unfortu-

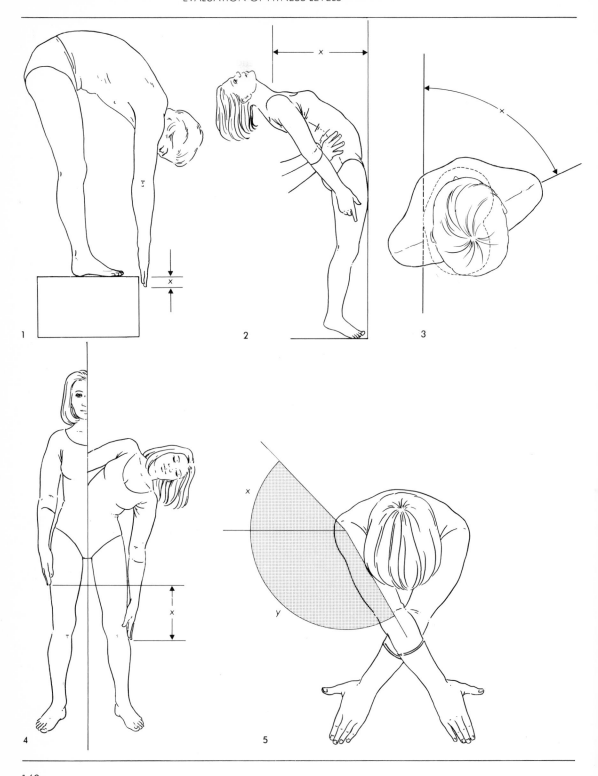

1

2

3

4

5

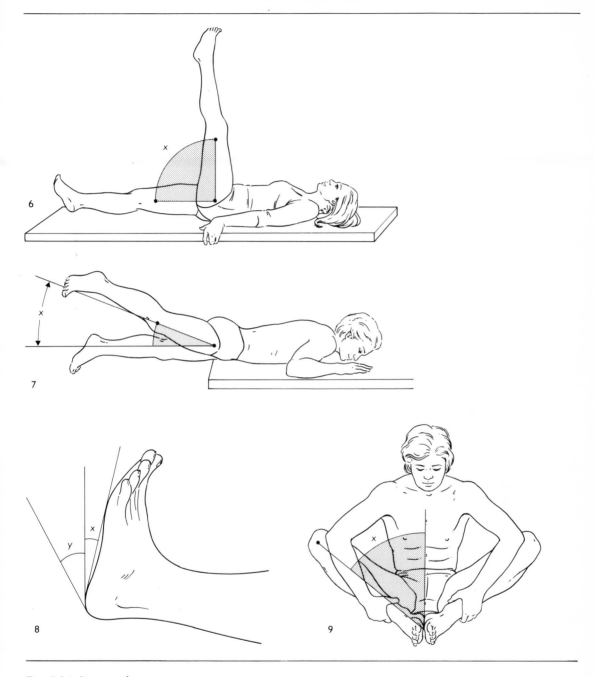

Fig. 5.14 Battery of flexibility tests (see text).

Fig. 5.15 Four measures of flexibility.

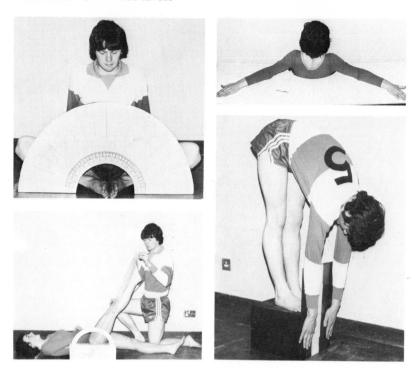

nately, even if the zero is correct this is no guarantee that other readings will be accurate. A set of scales must be calibrated over its entire working range with known weights. For more accurate measurements a beam balance is essential. The subject should stand upright and perfectly still, on the centre of the platform with his hands by his sides. The minimum of clothing should be worn; accurate measurements should be taken in the nude. In longitudinal studies try to take all measurements at the same time of day.

FAT CONTENT

There is no direct method of measuring the fat content of a living human but several indirect procedures are available. These vary widely in their complexity and accuracy and include: measurement of body density by weighing the individual in air and under water, body density from weight and body volume, estimation of muscle mass by counting the radiation from whole-body potassium, measurement of whole-body water from the dilution of tracer drugs or radio-isotopes, and estimations from anthropometric measurements. There are also a number of ways of measuring the thickness of the fat layer in various parts of the body. These include the use of X-rays, ultrasonics and skinfold calipers.

Estimation of body density by means of underwater weighing is the method most commonly used in research studies. The procedure is complicated by the need to estimate the volume of air in the subject's lungs at the time the weight is taken. This is a relatively complex process. Some writers appear to overestimate the precision of the underwater weighing method in relation to other techniques. Body density is not a direct measure of fat content and is influenced to some extent by variations in the density of the fat-free tissue. It is also difficult to measure with accuracy and unless the subject is accustomed to the procedure the results may be less reliable than those obtained from other methods of estimating fat. With inexperienced subjects the error may be $\pm$ 3 per cent of fat (Cureton *et al.* 1975) which is a percentage error of $\pm$ 15–20 per cent.

Fat content can be conveniently estimated from skinfold thicknesses. These are measured by taking a fold of flesh on a suitable site and measuring its thickness with calipers that exert a constant, standard pressure. Many investigators have produced equations for converting these measurements into an estimate of body density or percentage of fat. The number published must run into scores. When using these equations it is important to select one developed on subjects of the same race, sex and developmental status as the individuals to be tested.

The procedure described by Durnin and Rahaman (1967) may be used on subjects of both sexes and all ages although different equations are used for the computation of body density in the case of men, women, boys and girls. Skinfolds are measured on four sites: triceps, biceps, subscapular and supra-iliac. These sites are illustrated in Fig. 5.16.

Procedure for measuring skinfolds
1. Locate the site of measurement carefully, then mark it with a washable felt-tip pen. It has been shown that measurement errors are reduced when the sites are marked in advance of taking the measurements (Womersly and Durnin, 1973).

2. Grasp the skinfold between the thumb and forefinger of the left hand. Ensure that the fold is as large as possible and that it contains all the subcutaneous fat at the site of measurement.

3. Hold the fold between the finger and thumb of the left hand *while* the measurement is being taken.

4. Take the reading 2–5 seconds after the application of the caliper jaws.

5. Ensure that the skinfold is not distorted by pressure or tension from adjacent clothing.

With the Durnin and Rahaman procedure there are two steps in the conversion of skinfold thicknesses into an estimate of percentage fat:

(1) skinfold thickness $\rightarrow$ estimate of body density;
(2) body density $\rightarrow$ estimate of percentage fat.

Fig. 5.16 Body circumferences and skinfolds. Circumferences: (1) bideltoid; (2) lower thigh; (3) arm; (4) waist; (5) forearm; (6) thigh; (7) calf. Skinfolds: (a) biceps; (b) forearm; (c) supra-iliac; (d) abdominal; (e) front thigh; (f) triceps; (g) subscapular; (h) lower back; (i) buttocks; (j) rear thigh; (k) calf. The skinfolds should be raised at right angles to the direction of the arrow in the diagram, e.g. the abdominal skinfold is vertical.

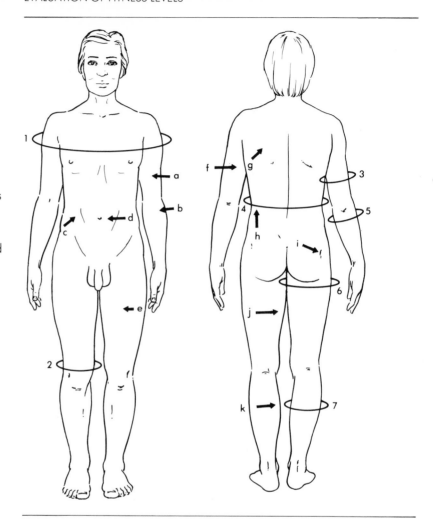

Conversion of skinfold thicknesses to an estimate of body density
The four skinfolds are added together and substituted in one of the following equations:

Men: body density = $1.161 - 0.0632 \log_{10}$(total skinfolds)
Women: body density = $1.1581 - 0.0720 \log_{10}$(total skinfolds)
Boys: body density = $1.1533 - 0.0643 \log_{10}$(total skinfolds)
Girls: body density = $1.1369 - 0.0598 \log_{10}$(total skinfolds)

Conversion of body density scores to an estimate of percentage fat
This equation is due to Siri (1956) and is the same for all types of subject:

$$\text{percentage fat} = \left(\frac{4.95}{\text{body density}} - 4.5 \right) \times 100$$

Example: For an adult male with skinfolds of 11.8, 12.6, 4.2, and 10.7 mm:

total skinfolds $= 39.3$ mm

body density $= 1.161 - 0.0632 \log_{10}(39.3)$
$= 1.0602$

therefore,

percentage fat $= \left(\dfrac{4.95}{1.0602} - 4.5 \right) \times 100$
$= 16.9$ per cent

When carried out by an experienced investigator the 95 per cent confidence limits of the estimate are within ± 6 per cent of fat (Cureton *et al.* 1975; Watson and O'Donovvan 1976b). The relationship with estimations made from direct measurements of body density is within ± 2 per cent of fat.

The Durnin and Rahaman method of estimating fat was developed for use with sedentary individuals and is not always ideal for use with sportsmen because of differences in the distribution of subcutaneous fat. The procedure described below was developed by the author for use with male athletes between the ages of 18 and 30. The use of over 20 skinfold sites was investigated and from these the six which related most closely to overall fat content and to anaerobic power output were selected. These skinfolds were on the abdomen, front thigh, triceps, buttocks, lower back and biceps. They are illustrated in Fig. 5.16.

Using these six skinfolds the percentage of fat can be estimated using the equation:

percentage fat $= 29.481 \log_{10}$ (sum of six skinfolds) $- 40.101$

Example: In a sportsman where the sum of the six skinfolds is 60 mm:

percentage fat $= 29.481 \log_{10}(60) - 40.101$
$= 29.481 \times 1.7782 - 40.101$
$= 12.32$ per cent

Fat-free weight

Fat-free weight is the weight of the whole body minus the weight of fat. It can be estimated by taking an accurate measurement of body weight and then subtracting the weight of fat.

Example: Individual of weight 72.65 kg; fat content 16.9 per cent:

weight of fat $= \dfrac{72.65 \times 16.9}{100} = 12.3$ kg

therefore,

fat-free weight $= 72.65 - 12.3$ kg
$= 60.4$ kg

Changes in body weight are influenced both by changes in fat-free weight and the fat content of the body. This is illustrated in Fig. 5.17.

Fig. 5.17 Changes in body weight, fat content and fat-free weight: (a) body weight remained constant due to the gain in fat-free weight being equal to the loss in fat content; (b) the rise in fat content was the same as the loss in fat-free weight and body weight again remained constant; (c) a loss in weight due to a reduction in fat content; (d) loss of fat but a greater increase in fat-free weight – the outcome of a successful training programme.

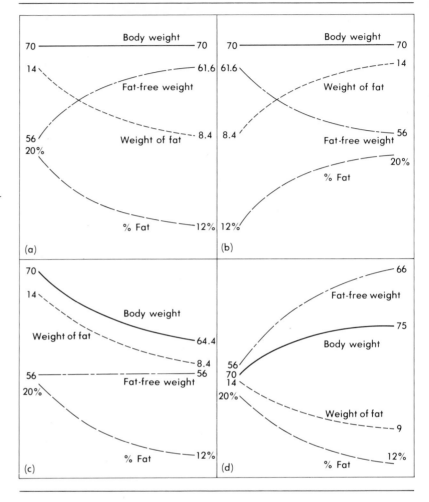

Other anthropometric measurements

Certain limb and trunk circumferences may be used as a guide to muscle development (see Fig. 5.16). Limb circumferences should first be converted to 'muscle plus bone' (M+B) sizes by allowing for the thickness of the layer of subcutaneous fat. Estimates of arm, forearm, thigh and calf (M+B) may be made using the equations:

arm (M+B) circum.   = arm circum. – 1.57(triceps + biceps)
forearm (M+B) circum. = forearm circum. – 1.57(forearm + 4)
thigh (M+B) circum.   = thigh circum. – 1.57(thigh front + thigh back)
calf (M+B) circum.   = calf circum. – 1.57(calf + 5)

The bracketed words indicate skinfold thickness as illustrated in Fig. 5.16. All measurements should be in millimetres.

Certain aspects of body shape can be quantified by expressing

Table 5.3 Anthropometric measurements expressed as raw scores and as a percentage of height. Mean and standard deviations* for 106 sportsmen

	Raw measurements		Percentage of height	
	Mean	S.D.	Mean	S.D.
Height (mm)	1,772	55	–	–
Weight (kg)	71.06	5.86	–	–
Sitting height (mm)	967	28	52.9	1.0
Biacromial diam. (mm)	410	13	23.1	0.7
Bi-iliac diam. (mm)	277	14	15.6	0.7
Humerus diam. (mm)	70.1	3.7	4.0	0.2
Femur diam. (mm)	96.2	4.2	5.4	0.2
Ankle diam. (mm)	76.5	3.6	4.3	0.2
Arm length (mm)	790	30	44.6	1.0
Femur length (mm)	398	24	22.5	1.2
Neck circum. (mm)	371	17	20.9	1.1
Bideltoid circum. (mm)	1,137	49	64.2	3.0
Arm circum. (mm)	282	18	15.9	1.2
Forearm circum. (mm)	268	13	15.1	0.8
Thigh circum. (mm)	554	28	31.3	1.8
Lower thigh circum. (mm)	382	30	21.6	1.5
Calf circum. (mm)	372	20	21.0	1.3
Skinfolds (mm)				
Triceps	7.8	2.2		
Biceps	4.3	0.8		
Abdominal	10.0	3.7		
Front thigh	9.7	2.6		
Lower back	12.2	5.2		
Buttocks	15.2	4.3		
Subscapular	9.4	1.8		
Supra-iliac	6.7	2.2		

* Approximately 68% of all observations lie within ± 1 standard deviations of the mean and 95% of observations lie within ± 2 standard deviations.

anthropometric widths, lengths and circumferences as a percentage of the subject's height. Mean values of a number of these ratios, together with the corresponding raw scores, are given in Table 5.3.

Body circumferences are influenced by bone lengths and widths and these sizes should be taken into account when assessing the muscle development of the sportsman. For example, bideltoid circumference, expressed as a percentage of that expected from bone sizes, is given by x, where:

$$x = 100 \text{ (bideltoid circum.)}/ (1.484 \text{ (biacromial diam.)} + 4.269 \text{ (ankle diam.)} + 205.227)$$

Example: If the bideltoid circumference is 1,200 mm when the biacromial and ankle diameters are, respectively, 410 and 76 mm, then:
$x = 105.4$ per cent
which means that the bideltoid circumference is 5.4 per cent greater than that expected from the athlete's bone sizes.

POSTURE

A subjective assessment of four aspects of posture, important in relation

Fig. 5.18 Anthropometric measurements.
(a) biacromial diameter
(b) thigh circumference
(c) arm length (d) femur length (e) abdominal skinfold (f) triceps skinfold
(g) humerus diameter
(h) femur diameter.

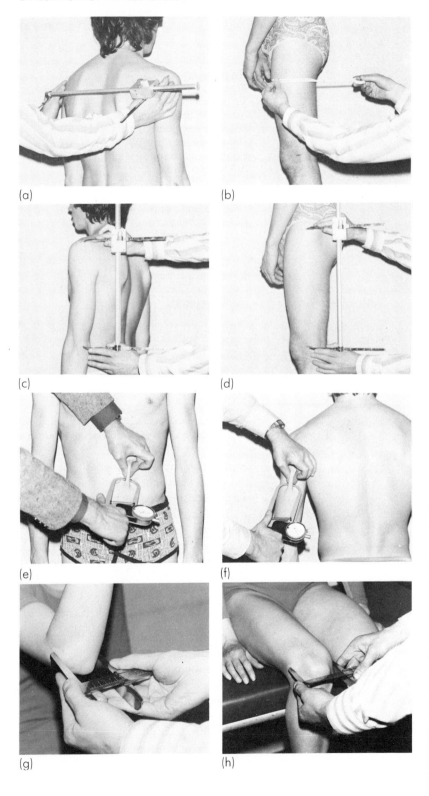

(a)

(b)

(c)

(d)

(e)

(f)

(g)

(h)

Fig. 5.19 Chart for assessment of four aspects of posture (see text).

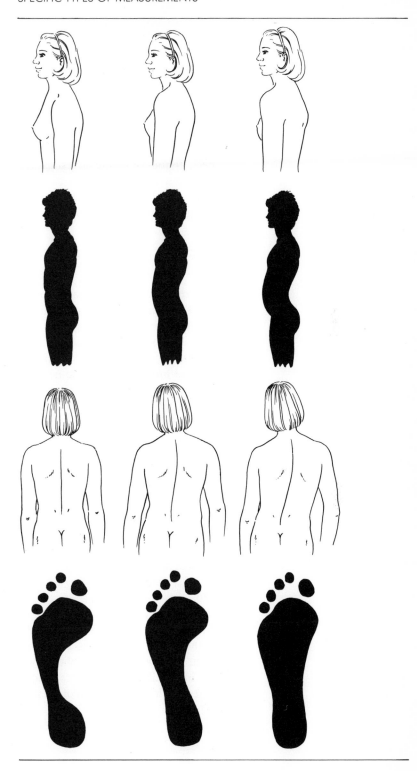

to physical performance, can be made using the chart illustrated in Fig. 5.19. In the case of the first three items a score of 5 indicates ideal posture, 3 a slight deviation from the ideal, and 1 a marked deviation.

In sportsmen the first two conditions illustrated in the diagram (abducted scapulae and lordosis, respectively) are likely to be due to muscle imbalance and can usually be corrected by means of a suitable exercise programme. The third (scoliosis) may also have this cause but can be due to a lateral curvature of the spine. An X-ray is required to determine this. Flat-feet (a score of 1 on the lower diagram) have been found by some investigators to be associated with an increased incidence of shin splints and foot pain, but very high arches (a score of 5) can also cause problems and may necessitate the use of specially designed running shoes or the wearing of an arch support.

THE INTERPRETATION OF TEST RESULTS

This requires considerable experience and skill as a large number of factors must be taken into account. Performance tests are influenced by invariable characteristics – age, gender, size, somatotype, motor unit distribution – and other genetic effects in addition to the athlete's state of training. As discussed in earlier chapters, genetic effects are frequently the dominant influence. It is also necessary to take into account the specificity of the test in relation to the athlete's competitive activity and the reliability of the measuring technique used.

Another problem lies in the definition of what is desirable in relation to any particular sport. Physical requirements are unique to each individual activity and there is an urgent need for the various sporting organisations to develop activity-specific evaluation procedures and to provide norms for them which take into account differences in the invariable characteristics listed above.

Some of the difficulties of interpretation are removed if the tests are repeated on the same subjects at regular intervals. The individual then acts as his own control and the influence of many of the invariable factors listed above can be eliminated, or considerably reduced. An example of a series of tests carried out on one individual is given in Fig. 5.20.

Longitudinal evaluation of test results is by far the most satisfactory procedure. Where this is not possible, such as after the first set of measurements are taken, it is better to compare the subject with his peers than with tables of published norms. Because of racial and other kinds of inter-subject differences, and systematic errors in measuring techniques, such data are often of very little value.

Fig. 5.20 Results of a series of clinical and laboratory tests on one field-game player. At the initial test in March it was found that lactic endurance was high but that knee extension strength was below average and fat content excessive. Clinical findings were normal except for knee instability. The athlete was given weight exercises to develop the quads and put on a programme of aerobic training in an attempt to bring the $\dot{V}_{O_2max}$ up to the level of his anaerobic endurance and to reduce fat content. By May the individual's fat content had dropped and knee extension strength had improved. But the flexion/extension ratio was now unsatisfactory and $\dot{V}_{O_2max}$ had dropped dramatically. The blood test results suggested that this may have been due to anaemia caused by folate and B_{12} deficiency. The athlete was advised to modify his diet and given vitamin and mineral supplements. He was also put on a wider range of leg exercises including some for the hamstrings. Subsequently the individual's clinical findings were all normal and his performance variables improved.

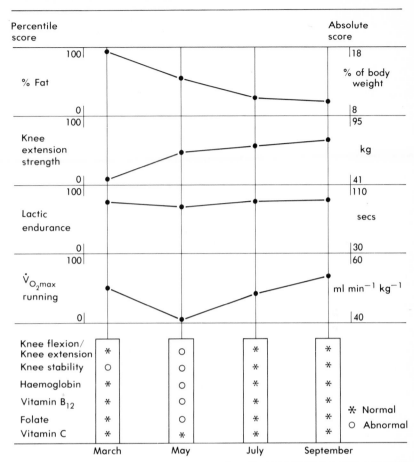

REFERENCES

Adams, G. M. and H. A. De Vries (1973) Physiological effects of an exercise training regimen upon women aged 52 to 79, *J. Geront.* **28**: 50–5

Ahlborg, G., L. Hagenfeldt and J. Wahren (1975) Substrate utilisation by the inactive leg during one-leg or arm exercise, *J. appl. Physiol.* **39**: 718–23

American Academy of Orthopaedic Surgeons (1965) *Joint Motion: Method of Measuring and Recording* (reprinted by the British Orthopaedic Association 1966), London: Churchill Livingston

Asmussen, E. and H. E. Christenssen (1967) *Kompendum i Legemsovelsernes Specielle Teori*, Kobenhavens Universites Fond til Tilverjbringelse af Lare-midler: Kobenhavn.

Asmussen, E. and B. Mazin (1978) A central nervous component in local muscular fatigue, *Europ. J. appl. Physiol.* **38**: 9–15

Astrand, P. O. (1967) Commentary, in Procedings of international symposium on physical activity and cardiovascular health, *Canad. Med. Ass. J.* **96**: 730

Astrand, P. O. and K. Rodahl (1970) *Text Book of Work Physiology*, New York: McGraw-Hill

Astrand, P. O. and I. Rhyming (1954) A nomogram for calculation of aerobic capacity (physical fitness) from pulse rate during sub-maximal work, *J. appl. Physiol.* **1**: 218–21

Atomi, Y., K. Ito, H. Iwasaki and M. Miyashita (1978) Effects of intensity and frequency of training on aerobic work capacity of young females, *J. Sports Med.* **18**: 3–9

Atomi, Y. and M. Miyashita (1974) Maximal aerobic power of Japanese active and sedentary adult females of different ages, *Med. Sci. Sports* **6**: 223–5

Baldwin, K. M., W. G. Cheadle, O. M. Martinez, and D. A. Cooke (1977) Effects of functional overload on enzyme levels in different types of skeletal muscle, *J. appl. Physiol.* **42**: 3.2–17

Baldwin, K. M., G. H. Klinkefuss, R. L. Terjung, P. A. Mole and J. O. Holloszy (1972) Respiratory capacity of red, white and intermediate muscle: adaptive response to exercise, *Am. J. Physiol* **222**: 373–8

Baldwin, K., W. W. Winder, R. L. Terjung and J. L. Holloszy (1973) Glycolytic enzymes in different types of muscle: adaptions to exercise, *Am. J. Physiol.* **225**: 962–6

Balke, B. and R. W. Ware (1959) An experimental study of physical fitness of Air Force personnel, *U.S. Armed Forces Med. J.* **10**: 675–88

Bar-Or, O., H. M. Lundegren and E. R. Buskirk (1969) Heat tolerance of exercising obese and lean women, *J. appl Physiol.* **26**: 403–309

Bar-Or, O. and L. D. Zwiren (1975) Maximum oxygen consumption test during arm exercise – reliability and validity, *J. appl. Physiol.* **38**: 424–6

Barnard, R. J., V. R. Edgerton and J. B. Peter (1970) Effects of exercise on skeletal muscle. I: Biochemical and histochemical properties, *J. appl. Physiol.* **28**: 762–6

Barnard, R. J. and J. B. Peter (1971) Effects of exercise on skeletal muscle. III: Cytochrome changes, *Am. J. Physiol.* **31**: 904–8

Baum, E., K. Bruck and H. P. Schwennicke (1976) Adaptive modifications in the thermoregulatory system of long-distance runners, *J. appl. Physiol.* **40**: 404–10

Belcastro, A. N. and A. Bonen (1975) Lactate removal rates during controlled and uncontrolled recovery exercise, *J. appl. Physiol.* **39**: 932–6

Benedict, F. G., and E. P. Cathcart (1913) *Muscular Work; a metabolic study with special reference to the efficiency of the human body as a machine*, Washington: Carnegie Institute

Benzi, G., P. Panceri, M. De Barnardi, R. Villa, E. Arcelli, L. d'Angelo, E. Arrigoni and F. Berte (1975) Mitochondrial enzyme adaption of skeletal muscle to endurance training, *J. appl. Physiol.* **38**: 565–9

Berger, R. (1962a) Effect of varied weight training programme on strength, *Res. Quart.* **33**: 329–33

Berger, R. (1962b) Optimum repetitions for the development of strength, *Res. Quart.* **33**: 334–8

Berger, R. (1963) Comparison between static training and various dynamic training programmes, *Res. Quart.* **34**: 131–5

Berger, R. (1965) Comparison of the effect of various weight training loads on strength, *Res. Quart.* **36**: 141–6

Bergh, H., A. Thorstensson, B. Sjodin, B. Hulten, K. Piehl and J. Karlsson (1978) Maximum oxygen uptake and muscle fibre types in trained and un-trained humans, *Med. Sci. Sports* **10**: 151–4

Bergstom, J., L. Hermansen, E. Hultman and B. Saltin (1967) Diet, muscle glycogen and endurance performance, *Acta Physiol. Scand.* **71**: 140–50

Billing, H. and E. Loewendahl (1949) *Mobilisation of the Human Body*, California: Stanford University Press

Binkhorst, R. A., L. Hoofd and A. C. A. Vissers (1977) Temperature and force–velocity relationship of human muscles, *J. appl. Physiol.* **42**: 471–5

Bonjer, F. N. (1966) Measurement of working capacity by assessment of the aerobic capacity in a single session, *Fed. Proc.* **25**: 1363–5

Bosco, C. and P. V. Komi (1979) Mechanical characteristics and fibre composition of human leg extensor muscles, *Europ. J. appl. Physiol.* **41**: 275–84

Bouchard, C., P. Godbout, J. C. Mondor and C. Leblanc (1979) Specificity of maximum aerobic power, *Europ. J. appl. Physiol.* **40**: 85–93

Brooke, C. G. D., R. M. C. Huntley and J. Slack (1975) Influence of heredity and environment in determination of the skinfold thickness of children, *Br. Med. J.* **2**: 719–21

Burke, E. R., F. Cerny, D. Costill and W. Fink (1977) Characteristics of skeletal muscle in competitive cyclists, *Med. Sci. Sports* **9**: 109–12

Burke, R. E. and V. R. Edgerton (1975) Motor unit properties and selective involvement in movement, in *Exercise and Sports Science Reviews*, Vol. III (eds J. H. Wilmore and J. F. Keogh), New York: Academic Press

Burkett, L. N. (1970) Causative factors in hamstring strains, *Med. Sci. Sports* **2**: 39–42

Carter, J. E. L. (1970) The somatotypes of athletes – a review, *Human Biology* **42**: 535–69

Chui, E. (1950) The effects of systematic weight training on athletic power, *Res. Quart.* **21**: 188–94

Clarke, D. and F. Henry (1961) Neuromuscular specificity and increased speed from strength development, *Res. Quart.* **32**: 315–25

Clarke, D. and G. Stull (1970) Endurance training as a determinant of strength and fatiguability, *Res. Quart.* **41**: 19–26

Costill, D. L. (1977a) Fluids for athletic performance: why and what should you drink during prolonged exercise, in *Towards an Understanding of Human Performance* (ed. E. J. Burke), New York: Mouvement Publications

Costill, D. L., E. F. Coyle, W. F. Fink, G. R. Lesmes and F. A. Witzmann (1979a) Adaptions in skeletal muscle following strength training, *J. appl. Physiol.* **46**: 96–9

Costill, D. L., J. Daniels, W. Evans, W. Fink, G. Krahenbuhl and B. Saltin (1976a) Skeletal muscle enzymes and fibre composition in male and female track athletes, *J. appl. Physiol.* **40**: 149–54

Costill, D. L., W. J. Fink, L. H. Getchell, J. L. Joy and F. A. Witzmann (1979b) Lipid metabolism in skeletal muscle of endurance-trained males and females, *J. appl. Physiol.* 40: 149–54

Costill, D. L., W. J. Fink and M. L. Pollock (1976b) Muscle fibre composition and enzyme activities of elite distance runners, *Med. Sci. Sports* **8**: 96–100

Costill, D. L. and B. Saltin (1974) Factors limiting gastric emptying during rest and exercise, *J. appl. Physiol.* **37**: 679–83

Cotes, J. E. (1965) *Lung Function: Assessment and Application in Medicine*, Oxford: Blackwell

Cotes, J. E., C. T. M. Davies, O. E. Edholm, M. J. R. Healey and J. M. Tanner (1969) Factors relating to the aerobic capacity of 46 British males and females aged 18–28 years, *Proc. R. Soc. Lond., Series B.* **174**: 91–114

Cotes, J. E. and R. F. Woolmer (1962) A comparison between 27 laboratories of the analysis of an expired air sample, *J. Physiol.* **163**: P37-7

Coyle, E. F., D. L. Costill and G. R. Lesmes (1979) Leg extensor power and muscle fibre composition, *Med. Sci. Sports* **11**: 12–15

Cureton, K. J., R. A. Boileau and T. G. Lohman (1975) A comparison of densiometric, potassium 40 and skinfold estimates of body composition in prepubescent boys, *Human Biology* **36**: 32–44

Cumming, G. R. and R. Danziger (1963) Bicycle ergometer studies in children, *Pediatrics* **32**: 202–8

Cumming, G. R., A. Goodwin, G. Baggley and J. Antel (1969) Repeated measurements of aerobic capacity during a week of intensive training at a youths track camp, *Canad. J. Physiol. Pharmacol.* **45**: 805–11

Cunningham, D. A. and J. A. Faulkner (1969) The effect of training on aerobic and anaerobic metabolism during a short exhaustive run, *Med. Sci. Sports* **1**: 65–9

Cunningham, D. A., D. McCrimmon and L. F. Vlach (1979) Cardiovascular response to interval and continuous training in women, *Europ. J. appl. Physiol.* **41**: 187–97

Daniels, J. and N. Oldbridge (1971) Changes in oxygen consumption in young boys during growth and running training, *Med. Sci. Sports* **3**: 161–5

Daniels, J., N. Oldbridge, F. Nagle and B. White (1978a) Differences and changes in $\dot{V}_{O_2}$ among young runners 10 to 18 years of age, *Med. Sci. Sports* **10**: 200–3

Daniels, J. T., R. A. Yarbrough and C. Foster (1978b) Changes in $\dot{V}_{O_2 max}$ and running performance with training, *Europ. J. appl. Physiol.* **39**: 249–54

Davies, C. T. M. (1968) Limitations to the prediction of maximum oxygen intake from cardiac frequency measurements, *J. appl. Physiol.* **24**: 700–6

Davies, C. T. M., C. A. Barnes and S. Godfrey (1972) Body composition and maximum exercise performance in children, *Human Biology* **44**: 195–214

Davies, C. T. M. and A. V. Knibbs (1971) The training stimulus – the effects of intensity, duration and frequency of effort on maximum aerobic power output, *Inter. Z. angew. Physiol.* **29**: 299–305

Davies, R. E. (1971) The dynamics of the energy rich phosphates, in *Limiting*

Factors of Physical Performance (ed. J. Keul), Stuttgard: Thieme

Davis, J. A. and V. A. Convertius (1975) A comparison of the heart rate methods for predicting endurance training intensity, *Med. Sci. Sports* **7**: 295–8

De Lateur, B., J. Lehmann and W. Fordyce (1968) A test of the De Lorme maxim, *Arch. Phys. Med. Rehabil.* **49**: 245–8

De Lorme, T. and A. Watkins (1948) Techniques of progressive resistance exercise, *Arch. Phys. Med. Rehabil.* **49**: 263–73

De Lorme, T. and A. Watkins (1951) *Progresssive Resistance Exercise*, New York: Appleton-Century-Crofts

De Vries, H. A. (1970) Physiological effects of an exercise training regimen upon men aged 52–88, *J. Geront.* **25**: 325–36

De Vries, H. A. (1974) *Physiology of Exercise for Physical Education and Athletics*, Iowa: Brown

Depocas, F., Y. Minaire and J. Chatonnet (1969) Rates of formation and oxidation of lactic acid in dogs at rest and during moderate exercise, *Canad. J. Physiol. Pharmacol.* **47**: 603–10

Dintiman, G. B. (1964) Effects of various training programmes on running speed, *Res. Quart.* **35**: 456–63

Drinkwater, B. L. and S. M. Horvath (1979) Heat tolerance and aging, *Med. Sci. Sports* **11**: 49–55

Durnin, J. V. G. A., J. M. Brockway and H. W. Whitcher (1960) Effects of a short period of training of varying severity on some measurements of physical fitness, *J. appl. Physiol.* **15**: 161–5

Durnin, J. V. G. A. and M. M. Rahaman (1967) The assessment of the amount of fat in the human body from measurements of skinfold thicknesses, *Br. J. Nutr.* **21**: 681–9

Eddy, D. O., L. L. Sparks and D. A. Adeliz (1977) The effects of continuous and interval training in women and men, *Europ. J. appl. Physiol.* **37**: 83–92

Edgerton, V. R. (1976) Neuromuscular adaptions to power and endurance work, *Canad. J. appl. Sports Sci.* **1**: 49–58

Edgerton, V. R., L. Gerchman and R. Carrow (1969) Histochemical changes in rat skeletal muscle after exercise, *Exp. Neurol.* **24**: 110–23

Ekblom, B. (1969) Effects of physical training on adolescent boys, *J. appl. Physiol.* **27**: 350–5

Ekblom, B., P. O. Astrand, B. Saltin, J. Stenberg, and B. Wallstom (1968) Effects of training on circulatory response to exercise, *J. appl. Physiol.* **24**: 518–28

Eriksson, B. O. (1969) Physical training, oxygen supply and muscle metabolism in 11–13 year old boys, *J. appl. Physiol.* **27**: 350–5

Eriksson, B., P. Gollnick and B. Saltin (1973) Muscle metabolism and enzyme activities after training in boys 11–13 years old, *Acta Physiol. Scand.* **87**: 485–97

Falch, D. K., and S. B. Strømme (1979) Pulmonary blood volume and interventricular circulation time in physically trained and untrained subjects, *Europ. J. appl. Physiol.* **40**: 211–8

Foster, C., D. L. Costill and W. J. Fink (1979) Effects of pre-exercise feeding on endurance performance, *Med. Sci. Sports* **11**: 1–5

Fox, E. L., R. L. Bartels, J. Klinzig and K. Ragg (1977) Metabolic responses to interval training of high and low power output, *Med. Sci. Sports* **9**: 191–6

Froelicher, V. F. Jr, H. Brammell, G. Davis, I. Noguera, A. Stewart and M. Lancaster (1974) A comparison of the reproducibility and physiologic response to three maximum treadmill exercise protocols, *Chest* **65**: 512–17

Gettman, L. R., J. J. Ayres, M. L. Pollock and A. Jackson (1978) The effects of circuit weight-training on strength, cardio-respiratory function and body composition of adult men, *Med. Sci. Sports* **10**: 171–6

Gisolfi, C. (1973) Work heat tolerance derived from interval training. *J. appl. Physiol.* **35**: 349–54

Glassford, R. G., G. H. Y. Baycroft, A. W. Sedgwick and R. B. J. MacNab (1965) Comparison of maximal oxygen uptake values determined by predicted and actual methods, *J. appl. Physiol.* **20**: 509–13

Glenhill, N. and R. B. Eynon (1972) The intensity of training, in *Training Scientific Basis and Application* (ed. A. W. Taylor), Springfield, Ill.: Thomas, Chapter 8.

Goldfuss, A. J., C. A. Morehouse and B. F. Le Veau (1973) Effect of muscular tension on knee stability, *Med. Sci. Sports* **5**: 267–71

Gollnick, P., R. Armstrong, B. Saltin, C. Saubert, W. Sembrowich and R. Shephard (1973) Effects of training on enzyme activity and fibre composition of human skeletal muscle, *J. appl. Physiol.* **34**: 107–11.

Gollnick, P. D., R. B. Armstrong, C. W. Saubert IV, K. Piehl and B. Saltin (1972) Enzyme activity and fibre composition in skeletal muscle of untrained and trained men, *J. appl. Physiol.* **33**: 312–9

Gollnick, P. and D. King (1969) Effect of exercise and training on mitochondria of rat skeletal muscle, *Am. J. Physiol.* **216**: 1502–9

Guth, L. (1968) 'Trophic' influences of nerve on muscle, *Physiol. Rev.* **48**: 645–87

Guyton, A. C. (1963) *Cardiac Output and its Regulation*, Philadelphia: Saunders

Guyton, A. C. (1966) *Textbook of Medical Physiology*, Philadelphia: Saunders

Guyton, A. C. (1968) Regulation of cardiac output, *Anesthesiology* **29**: 314

Guyton, A. C., G. G. Armstrong Jr and P. L. Chipley (1956) Pressure–volume curves of the entire arterial and venous system in the living animal, *Am. J. Physiol.* **179**: 261

Hagermann, F. C., M. D. McKirnan and J. A. Pompei (1975) Maximum oxygen consumption of conditioned and unconditioned oarsmen, *J. Sports. Med.* **15**: 43–8

Hamilton, P. and G. M. Andrews (1976) Influence of growth and athletic training on heart and lung functions, *Europ. J. appl. Physiol.* **36**: 27–38

Haymers, E. M., R. J. McCormick and E. R. Buskirk (1975) Heat tolerance of exercising lean and obese pre-pubertal boys, *J. appl. Physiol.* **39**: 475–61

Helgheim, I., Ø. Hetland, S. Nilsson, F. Ingjer and S. B. Strømme (1979) The effects of vitamin E on serum enzyme level following heavy exercise, *Europ. J. appl. Physiol.* **40**: 283–9

Hellebrandt, F. A. (1958) Application of the overload principle to muscle training in man, *Am. J. Phys. Med.* **37**: 278–83

Henane, R., R. Flandrois and J. P. Charbonnier (1977) Increase in sweating sensitivity by endurance conditioning in man, *J. appl. Physiol.* **43**: 822–8

Hermansen, L., E. Hultman and B. Saltin (1967) Muscle glycogen during prolonged severe exercise, *Acta Physiol. Scand.* **71**: 129–39

Hermansen, L. and O. Vaage (1977) Lactate disappearance and glycogen synthesis in human muscle after maximal exercise, *Am. J. Physiol.* **223**: 422–9

Hickson, R. C. (1980) Interference of strength development by simultaneously training for strength and endurance, *Europ. J. appl. Physiol.* **45**: 255–63

Hickson, R. C., J. M. Hagberg, R. K. Conlee, D. A. Jones, A. A. Ehsani and W. W. Winder (1979) Effects of training on hormonal response to exercise in competitive swimming, *Europ. J. appl. Physiol.* **41**: 211–19

Hickson, R. C., W. W. Heusner, and W. D. Van Huss (1976) Skeletal muscle enzyme alterations after sprint and endurance training, *J. appl. Physiol.* **40**: 868–72

Hislop, H. J. (1963) Quantitative changes in human muscular strength during isometric exercise, *J. Am. Phys. Ther. Assoc.* **43**: 21–38

Holloszy, J. O. (1967) Biochemical changes in muscle; effects of exercise on mitochondrial oxygen uptake and respiratory enzyme activity, *J. Biol.*

Chem. **242**: 2278–82

Houston, M. E. and J. A. Thomson (1977) The response of endurance adapted adults to intense anaerobic training, *Europ. J. appl. Physiol.* **36**: 207–13

Hultman, E. and J. Bergstom (1967) Muscle glycogen synthesis in relation to diet, studied in normal subjects, *Acta Med. Scand.* **82**: 109–17

Ikai, M. and A. Steinhaus (1961) Some factors modifying the expression of human strength, *J. appl. Physiol.* **16**: 157–63

Ingjer, F. (1979) Capillary supply and mitochondrial content of different skeletal muscle fibre types in untrained and endurance trained man. A histochemical and ultrastructural study, *Europ. J. appl. Physiol.* **40**: 197–209

Ingjer, F. and S. B. Strømme (1979) The effects of active, passive or no warm-up on the physiological response to heavy exercise, *Eurp. J. appl. Physiol.* **40**: 273–82

Issekutz, B., W. A. Shaw and A. C. Issekutz (1976) Lactate metabolism in resting and exercising dogs, *J. appl. Physiol.* **40**: 312–19

Jackson, J. H., B. J. Sharkey and L. Johnson (1968) Cardio-respiratory adaptions to training at specified frequencies, *Res. Quart.* **39**: 295–300

Johns, R. and V. Wright (1962) Relative importance of various tissues in joint stiffness, *J. appl. Physiol.* **17**: 824–8

Johnson, B. L. (1972) Eccentric vs. concentric training for strength development, *Med. Sci. Sports* **4**: 111–15

Johnson, B. L., J. W. Adamczyk, K. O. Tennoe and S. B. Strømme (1976) A comparison of concentric and eccentric muscle training, *Med. Sci. Sports* **8**: 35–8

Jorfeldt, L., A. Juhlin-Dannfelt, and J. Karlsson (1978) Lactate release in relation to tissue lactate in human skeletal muscle during exercise, *J. appl. Physiol.* **44**: 350–2

Karlson, P. (1968) *Introduction to Modern Biochemistry*, p. 79, New York: Academic Press

Karlsson, J., L. Nordesjo, L. Jorfeldt, and B. Saltin (1972) Muscle lactate, ATP and CP levels during exercise after physical training in man, *J. appl. Physiol.* **33**: 199–203

Karlsson, J. and B. Saltin (1971) Diet, muscle glycogen and endurance performance, *J. appl. Physiol.* **31**: 203–6

Karnoven, J. J., E. Kentala and O. Mustula (1957) The effects of training on heart rate: a longitudinal study, *Ann. Med. Expt. Biol. Fenn.* **35**: 307–15

Kavanagh, T., R. Shephard and V. Pandit (1974) Marathon running after myocardial infarction, *J. Am. Med. Assoc.* **229**: 1602–5

Kearne, J. T., G. A. Stull, J. L. Ewing Jr and J. W. Strein (1976) Cardio-respiratory responses of sedentary women as a function of training intensity, *J. appl. Physiol.* **41**: 822–5

Keul, J., E. Doll and D. Keppler (1972) *Energy Metabolism in Human Muscle*, Basel: Karger

Khosla, T. (1978) Standards on age, height and weight in olympic running events for men, *Br. J. Sports Med.* **12**: 97–101

Kilbom, A. (1971) Effect on women of physical training with low intensities, *Scand. J. Clin. Lab. Invest.* **28**, Supplement 119

Kindermann, W., G. Simon and J. Keul (1979) The significance of the aerobic – anaerobic transition for the determination of work load intensities during endurance training, *Europ. J. appl. Physiol.* **42**: 25–34

Klissouras, V. (1971) Hereditability of adaptive variation, *J. appl. Physiol.* **3**: 338–46

Klissouras, V. (1973) Prediction of potential performance with special reference to heredity, *J. Sports. Med.* **13**: 100–7

Knowlton, R. G. and D. S. Miles (1978) Metabolic response of untrained individuals to warm-up, *Europ. J. appl. Physiol.* **40**: 1–5

Knutten, H. G. (1967) Aerobic capacity of adolescents, *J. appl. Physiol.* **22**: 655–8

Komi, P. V. and E. R. Buskirk (1972) Effects of concentric and eccentric muscle conditioning on tension and electrical activity of human muscle, *Ergonomics* **15**: 417–34

Komi, P. V., J. T. Viitasalo, R. Rauramaa and V. Vihko (1978) Effects of isometric strength training on mechanical, electrical and metabolic aspects of muscle function, *Europ. J. appl. Physiol.* **40**: 45–55

Kral, J. (1974) The medical examination, in *Fitness Health and Work Capacity: Internation Standards for Assessment* (ed. L. A. Larson), London and New York: Macmillan

Kraus, H. and W. Raab (1961) *Hypokinetic Disease*, Illinois: Thomas

Lavine, R. L., D. T. Lowenthal, M. D. Gellman, S. Kline, L. R. Recant and L. I. Rose (1980) The effect of long-distance running on plasma immunoreactive glucogen levels, *Europ. J. appl. Physiol.* **43**: 41–4

Lawrance, J. P., R. C. Bower, W. P. Riehl and U. L. Smith (1975) Effects of tocopherol acetate on the swimming endurance of trained swimmers, *Am. J. Clin. Nutr.* **28**: 205–8

Leighton, J. R. (1942) A simple and reliable measure of flexibility, *Res. Quart.* **13**: 205

Leighton, J. (1957a) Flexibility characteristics of four specialised groups of college athletes, *Arch. Phys. Med. Rehabil.* **38**: 24–8

Leighton, J. (1957b) Flexibility characteristics of three groups of champion athletes, *Arch. Phys. Med. Rehabil.* **38**: 580–3

Lesmes, G. R., D. H. Costill, E. Coyle and W. J. Fink (1978a) Muscle strength and power changes during maximal isokinetic training, *Med. Sci, Sports* **10**: 266–9

Lesmes, G. R., E. L. Fox, C. Stevens and R. Otto (1978b) Metabolic response of females to high intensity interval training, *Med. Sci. Sports* **10**: 229–32

Magel, J. R., G. F. Foglia, W. D. McCardle, B. Gutin, G. S. Pechar and F. I. Katch (1975) Specificity of swim training on maximum oxygen uptake, *J. appl. Physiol.* **38**: 151–5

Maher, J. T., G. Beller, J. M. Foster and L. H. Hartley (1978) Radiographic changes in cardiac dimensions during exhaustive exercise in man, *J. Sports Med.* **18**: 263–69

Malarecki, I. (1954) Investigation on physiological justification of so-called 'warming-up', *Acta Physiol. Pol.* **5**: 543–6

Man, S. F. P. and N. Zamel (1976) Genetic influence on normal variability of maximum expiratory flow curves, *J. appl. Physiol.* **41**: 874–7

Margaria, R., I. Aghemo and E. Rovelli (1966) Measurement of muscular power (anaerobic) in man, *J. appl. Physiol.* **21**: 1662–4

Margaria, R., P. Cerretelli, and F. Mangili (1964) Kinetics and mechanism of oxygen debt contraction in man, *J. appl. Physiol.* **19**: 623–8

Margaria, R., H. T. Edwards and D. B. Dill (1933) The possible mechanism of contracting and paying the oxygen debt and the role of lactic acid in muscular contraction, *Am. J. Physiol.* **106**: 687–715

Margaria, R., R. V. Oliva, P. E. di Prampero and P. Cerretelli (1969) Energy utilisation in intermittent exercise of supra-maximal intensity, *J. appl. Physiol.* **26**: 752–6

Marks, J. (1968) *The Vitamins in Health and Disease: a Modern Reappraisal*, London: Churchill

Martin, B. R., S. Robinson, D. L. Wiegman and L. H. Anlick (1975) Effects of warm-up on metabolic responses to strenuous exercise, *Med. Sci. Sports* **7**: 146–9

Masley, J., A. Hairabedian and D. Donaldson (1953) Weight training in relation to speed, strength and coordination, *Res. Quart.* **24**: 308–15

Mathews, D. K. and E. L. Fox (1976) *The Physiological Basis of Physical Education and Athletics*, Philadelphia: Saunders

Mathews, D. K. and R. Kruse (1957) Effects of isometric and isotonic exercise on elbow flexor muscles, *Res. Quart.* **28**: 26–37

Mayer, J. (1953) Genetic, traumatic and environmental factors in obesity, *Physiol. Rev.* **33**: 472–508

Meyerhof, O. (1920) Uber die Energieumwandlungen im Muskel. II: Das Schicksol der Milchsaure in der Erholung-speriode des Muskels, *Pfluegers Arch.* **182**: 284–317

Meyerhof, O. (1922) Die Energieumwandlungen im Muskel. VI: Uber den Ursprung der Kontraktionswarme, *Pfluegers Arch.* **195**: 22–74

Milner-Brown, H. S , R. B. Stein and R. Yemm (1973) The orderly recruitment of human motor units during voluntary isometric contractions, *J. Physiol.* **230**: 359–70

Minaire, Y. (1973) Origine et destinée du lactate plasmatique, *J. Physiol.* (*Paris*) **66**: 229–57

Minard, D., H. S. Belding and J. R. Kingston (1957) Prevention of heat casualties, *J. Am. Med. Assoc.* **165**: 1813–18

Mitchell, J. H., B. M. Sproule and C. Chapman (1958) The physiological meaning of the maximum oxygen uptake test, *J. Clin. Invest.* **37**: 538–47

Moffatt, R. J., B. A. Stamford and R. D. Neill (1977) Placement of tri-weekly training sessions: importance regarding enhancement of aerobic capacity, *Res. Quart.* **48**: 583–91

Mole, P. A. and J. Holloszy (1970) Exercise induced increase in the capacity of skeletal muscle for palmitate, *Proc. Soc. Expt. Biol. Med.* **134**: 788–92

Mole, P. A., L. B. Oscai and J. O. Holloszy (1971) Adaptions of muscle to exercise, *J. Clin. Invest.* **50**: 2323–30

Montoye, H. J., H. L. Metzner and J. B. Keller (1975) Familial aggregation of strength and heart rate response to exercise, *Human Biology* **47**: 17–36

Morehouse, C. (1967) Development and maintenance of isometric strength of subjects with diverse initial strength, *Res. Quart.* **38**: 449–56

Morgan, R. E. and G. T. Adamson (1961) *Circuit Training* (2nd edn), London: Bell

Müller, E. A. (1959) Training muscle strength, *Ergonomics* **2**: 216–23

Müller, E. A. (1970) Influence of training and inactivity on muscle strength, *Arch. Phys. Med. Rehabil.* **51**: 449–62

Müller, E. A. and T. Hettinger (1954) Die Bedeutung der Trainingsgeschwindigkeit atrophierter von Muskeln, *Arbeitsphysiol.* **15**: 223–30

Müller, E. A. and W. Rohmert (1963) The speed increase of muscle strength through isometric exercise, *Inter Angew. Physiol.* **19**: 403–19

McArdle, W. D., J. R. Magel, D. J. Dekio, M. Toner and J. M. Chase (1978) Specificity of run training on $\dot{V}_{O_2max}$ and heart rate changes during running and swimming, *Med. Sci. Sports* **10**: 16–20

McCafferty, W. B. and S. M. Horvath (1977) Specificity of exercising and training: a sub-cellular review, *Res. Quart.* **48**: 358–71

McCormack, R. J. and E. R. Buskirk (1974) Heat tolerance of exercising lean and obese middle-aged men, (*Abstract*) *Fed. Proc.* **33**: 441

MacDougall, J. D., G. C. B. Elder, D. G. Sale, J. R. Moraz and J. R. Sutton (1980) Effects of strength training and immobilisation on human muscle fibres, *Europ. J. appl. Physiol.* **43**: 25–34

MacDougall, J. D., G. R. Ward, D. G. Sale and J. R. Sutton (1977) Biochemical adaption of human skeletal muscle to heavy resistance training and immobilisation, *J. appl. Physiol.* **43**: 700–3

McMorris, R. and E. Elkins (1954) A study of production and evaluation of muscular hypertrophy, *Acta Phys. Med. Rehabil.* **35**: 420–6

Nadel. E. R. (ed.) (1977) *Problems with Temperature Regulation during exercise,*

New York: Academic Press

Nadel, E. R. (1979) Control of sweating rate while exercising in the heat, *Med. Sci. Sports* **11**: 31–5

Nafstad, I. and S. Tollersrud (1970) The vitamin E deficiency syndrome in pigs, *Acta Vet. Scand.* **11**: 452–80

Nishiitsutsuji-Uwo, J. M. B. D. Ross and H. A. Krebs (1967) Metabolic activities of the isolated perfused rat kidney, *Biochem. J.* **103**: 852–62

O'Donoghue, D. H. (1970) *Treatment of Injuries to Athletes*, Philadelphia: Saunders

O'Hara, W. J., C. Allen and R. J. Shephard (1977) Loss of body weight and fat during exercise in a cold chamber, *Europ. J. appl. Physiol.* **37**: 205–18

O'Hara, W. J., C. Allen, R. J. Shephard and G. Allen (1979) Fat loss in the cold – a controlled study, *J. appl. Physiol.* **46**: 872–8

Osbourne, R. H., and F. V. De George (1959) *Genetic Basis of Morphological Variation*, Cambridge, Mass: Harvard University Press

Paul, P. and W. Holmes (1975) Free fatty acid and glucose metabolism during increased energy expenditure and after training, *Med. Sci. Sports* **7**: 176–84

Pendersen, P. and K. Jorgensen (1978) Maximal oxygen uptake in young women with training inactivity and retraining, *Med. Sci. Sports* **10**: 233–7

Perrine, J. J. and V. R. Edgerton (1978) Muscle force–velocity and power–velocity relationships under isokinetic loading, *Med. Sci. Sports* **10**: 159–66

Peter, J. B., S. Sawaki, R. J. Barnard, R. J. Edgerton and C. A. Gillespie (1971) Lactate dehydrogenase isoenzymes: distribution in fast-twitch red, fast-twitch white and slow-twitch intermediate fibres of guinea pig skeletal muscle, *Arch. Biochem. Biophys.* **144**: 304–7

Peterson, J. A. (1975) Total conditioning: a case study, *Athletic J.* **55**: 40–55

Pette, D., M.E. Smith, W. H. Staudte, and G. Vribova (1973) Effects of long term electrical stimulation on some contractile and metabolic characteristics of fast rabbit muscles, *Pfluegers Arch.* **338**: 257–72

Pettengale, P. and J. Holloszy (1967) Augmentation of skeletal muscle myoglobin by a programme of treadmill running, *Am. J. Physiol.* **213**: 783–5

Piehl, K. (1974) Time course for refilling glycogen stores in human muscle fibres following exercise-induced glycogen depletion, *Acta Physiol. Scand.* **90**: 297–302

Pipes, T. V. (1978) Variable resistance versus constant resistance strength training in adult males, *Europ. J. appl. Physiol.* **39**: 27–35

Pipes, T. V. and J. Wilmore (1975) Isokinetic vs. isotonic training in adult men, *Med. Sci. Sports* **7**: 262–74

Pollock, M. L. (1973) The quantification of endurance training programmes, in *Exercise and Sports Science Reviews*, Vol. I (ed. J. H. Wilmore), New York: Academic Press

Pollock, M. L., T. K. Cureton and L. Greniger (1969) Effects of frequency of training on working capacity, cardiovascular function and body composition in adult men, *Med. Sci. Sports* **1**: 70–4

Pollock, M. L., J. Dimmock, H. Miller, Z. Kendrick and A. Linnerud (1975) Effects of mode of training on cardiovascular function and body composition of adult men, *Med. Sci. Sports* **7**: 139–45

Pollock, M. L., L. A. Gettman, C. A. Milesis, M. D. Bah, L. Durstine and R. M. Johnson (1977) Effects of frequency and duration of training on attrition and incidence of injury, *Med. Sci. Sports* **9**: 31–6

Poortmans, J. R., J. D. Bossche and R. Leclercq (1978) Lactate uptake by inactive forearm during progressive leg exercise, *J. appl. Physiol.* **45**: 835–9

Poortsmans, J. R. and R. W. Jeanloz (1978) Quantitative immunological determination of 12 plasma proteins excreted in human urine collected before and after exercise, *J. Clin Invest.* **47**: 386–93

Prendergast, D. (1979) Aerobic and glycolytic metabolism in arm exercise, *J.*

appl. Physiol. **47**: 754–760

Ragg, K. E. (1979) Continuous and interval training programme influences upon leg speed, *J. Sports Med.* **19**: 157–64

Ramsey, J. M. and S. W. Pipoly Jr (1979) Response of erythrocyte 2, 3-diphosphoglycerate to strenuous exercise, *Europ. J. appl. Physiol.* **40**: 227–33

Rasch, P. J. (1971) Isometric exercise and gains of muscle strength, in *Frontiers of Fitness* (ed. R. J. Shephard), Springfield, Ill.: Thomas Rasch, P. J., J. W. Hamby and H. J. Burns Jr (1969) Protein dietary supplementation and physical performance, *Med. Sci. Sports* **1**: 195–9

Rasch, P. J. and E. L. Morehouse (1957) Effect of static and dynamic exercises on muscular strength and hypertrophy, *J. appl. Physiol.* **11**: 29–34

Recommended Dietary Allowances (1968) 7th revised edn, Washington D.C.: National Academy of Sciences

Roberts, A. D. and A. R. Morton (1978) Total and alactic oxygen debts after supra-maximal work, *Europ. J. appl. Physiol.* **38**: 281–9

Robinson, S., D. B. Dill, R. D. Robinson, S. P. Tzankoff and J. A. Wagner (1976) Physiological ageing of champion runners, *J. appl. Physiol.* **41**: 46–51

Roskamm, H. (1967) Optimum patterns of exercise for healthy adults, *Canad. Med. Assoc. J.* **96**: 895–899

Rowell, L. B. (1974) Human cardiovascular adjustments to exercise and thermal stress, *Physiol. Rev.* **54**: 75–157

Rudermann, N. E. (1975) Muscle amino acid metabolism and gluconeogensis, *Ann. Rev. Med.* **26**: 245–58

Rusko, H., M. Havu and E. Karvinen (1978) Aerobic capacity in Athletes, *Europ. J. appl. Physiol.* **38**: 151–9

Salmons, S. and G. Vrbova (1969) The influence of activity on some contractile characteristics of mammalian fast and slow twitch muscles, *J. Physiol.* **201**: 535–49

Saltin, B. and J. Stenberg (1964) Circulatory response to prolonged severe exercise, *J. appl. Physiol.* **19**: 833–8

Scheel, K., W. Herzog, G. Ritthaler, A. Wirth and H. Weicker (1979) Metabolic adaption to prolonged exercise, *Europ. J. appl. Physiol.* **41**: 101–8

Schickele, E. (1947) Environment and fatal heat stroke, *Military Surg.* **100**: 235–56

Scripture, E. Q., T. L. Smith and E. M. Brown (1894) On the education of muscular control and power, *Studies of Yale Psychology Laboratory* **2**: 114–19

Seleger, V., L. Dolejas, V. Karas and I. Pachlonnikova (1968) Adaption of trained athletes energy expenditure to repeat concentric and eccentric muscle contractions, *Inter. Z. angew. Physiol. einschl. Arbeitsphysiol.* **26**: 227–34

Sharkey, B. J. (1970) Intensity, duration and frequency and the development of cardiorespiratory endurance, *Med. Sci. Sports* **2**: 197–202

Sharman, I. M., M. G. Down and N. G. Norgan (1976) The effect of vitamin E on physiological function and athletic performance of trained swimmers, *J. Sports Med.* **16**: 215–25

Shaver, L. G. (1975) Cross transfer effects of conditioning and de-conditioning on muscular strength, *Ergonomics* **18**: 9–16

Sheldon, W. H. (1940), with S. S. Stevens and W. B. Tucker, *The Varieties of Human Physique*, New York: Harper

Sheldon, W. H. (1954), with C. W. Dupertuis and E. Mc Dermott, *Atlas of Men*, New York: Harper

Shephard, R. J. (1968) Intensity, duration and frequency of exercise as determinants of the response to a training programme, *Inter. Z. angew. Physiol.* **26**: 272–8

Shephard, R. J. (1969) *Endurance Fitness*, Toronto: University of Toronto Press

Shephard, R. J. (1971) The oxygen conductance equation, in *Frontiers of Fitness* (ed. R. J. Shephard), Springfield, Ill.: Thomas

Shephard, R. J. (1977) Programs of physical activity for the primary school – needless or a necessity?, in *Towards an Understanding of Human Performance* (ed. E. J. Burke), Ithaca, New York: Mouvement Publications

Shephard, R. J., R. Campbell, P. Pimm, D. Stuart and G. R. Wright (1974) Vitamin E, exercise and the recovery from physical activity, *Europ. J. appl. Physiol.* **33**: 119–26

Shields, J. (1962) *Monozygotic twins brought up apart and brought up together: an investigation into the genetic and environmental causes of variation in personality*, London: Oxford University Press.

Shire, T. L., J. P. Avallone, R. Boileau, T. H. Lohman and J. C. Wirth (1977) Effects of high-resistance and low-resistance bicycle ergometer training in college women on cardiorespiratory function and body composition, *Res. Quart.* **48**: 391–400

Siri, W. E. (1956) *Advances in Biological and Medical Physics* (eds J. H. Lawrence and C. A. Tobias), New York: Academic Press

Smith, D. P. and F. W. Stansky (1976) The effect of training and detraining on the body composition and cardiovascular response of young women to exercise, *J. Sports Med.* **16**: 112–20

Sorani, R. (1966) *Circuit Training*, Dubuque, Iowa: Brown

Sprynarova, S. (1966) Development of the relationship between aerobic capacity and the circulatory and respiratory reaction to moderate activity in boys 11 to 13 years, *Physiol. Bohemoslov* **15**: 253–64

Stamford, A. B., R. J. Moffatt, A. Weltman, C. Maldonado and M. Curtis (1978) Blood lactate disappearance after supra-maximal one-leg exercise, *J. appl. Physiol.* **45**: 244–8

Staudte, H. W. G. Exner and D. Pette (1973) Effects of short-term high-intensity (spirit) training on some contractile and metabolic characteristics of fast and slow muscle of the rat, *Pfluegers Arch.* **344**: 159–68

Strømme, S. B., F. Ingjer and H. D. Meen (1977) Assessment of maximum aerobic power in specifically trained athletes, *J. appl. Physiol.* **42**: 833–7

Stull, G. and D. Clarke (1970) High-resistance low-repetition training as a determiner of strength and fatiguability, *Res. Quart.* **41**: 105–9

Suominen, H., E. Heikkinen, H. Liesen, D. Michel and W. Hollmann (1977) Effects of 8 weeks endurance training on skeletal muscle metabolism in 56–70 year old sedentary men, *Europ. J. appl. Physiol.* **37**: 173–80

Tanner, J. M. (1952) The effect of weight-training on physique, *Am. J. Phys. Anthrop.*, N.S. **10**: 427–61

Tanner, J. M. (1964) *The Physique of the Olympic athlete*, London: Allen & Unwin

Taylor, H. L., E. Buskirk and A. Henschell (1955) Maximum oxygen uptake as an objective measure of cardiovascular performance, *J. appl. Physiol.* **8**: 73–80

Thistle, H., H. Hislop. M. M. Affroid and E. Lowman (1967) Isokinetic contraction: a new concept of resistive exercise, *Arch. Phys. Med. Rehabil.* **48**: 279–82

Thorstensson, A., G. Grimby, and J. Karlsson (1976) Force–velocity relationship and fibre composition in human knee extensor muscle, *J. appl. Physiol.* **40**: 12–6

Thorstensson, A., L. Larsson, P. Tesch and J. Karlsson (1977) Muscle strength and fibre composition in athletes and sedentary men, *Med. Sci. Sports* **9**: 26–30

Thorstensson, A., B. Sjodin and J. Karlsson (1975) Enzyme activities and muscle strength after sprint training in man, *Acta Physiol. Scand.* **94**: 313–18

Venerando, V. and M. Milani-Comaretti (1970) Twin studies in sport and physical performance, *Acta Gen. Med. Gemel.* **19**: 80–2

Vihko, V. J. Soimajarvi, E. Karvinen, P. Rahkila and M. Havu (1978) Lipid metabolism during exercise. I: Physiological characterisation of normal healthy subjects in relation to their physical fitness, *Europ. J. appl. Physiol.* **39**: 209–18

Vihko, V., A. Salminen and J. Rantamaki (1979) Exhaustive exercise, endurance training, and acid hydrolase activity in skeletal muscle, *J. appl. Physiol.* **47**: 43–50

Warmolts, J. R. and W. K. Engel (1973) Correlation of motor unit behaviour with histochemical myofibre type in humans by open-biopsy electromyography, in *New Developments in Electromyography and Clinical Neurophysiology*, Vol. 1 (ed. J. E. Desmedt), Basel: Karger

Watson, A. W. S. (1973) Weight changes during prolonged exercise, *Br. J. Sports Med.* **7**: 338–9

Watson, A. W. S. (1974) Lumbar lordosis and strain of the iliopsoas, *Br. J. Sports Med.* **8**: 203–4

Watson, A. W. S. (1978) Assessment of the cardiovascular fitness of sportsmen *J. Sports Med.* **18**: 193–200

Watson, A. W. S. (1979) A three year study of the effects of exercise on active young men, *Europ. J. appl. Physiol.* **40**: 107–15

Watson, A. W. S. (1982) Factors predisposing to sports injury in schoolboy rugby players, *J. Sports Med.* **21**: 417–22

Watson, A. W. S. (1983) Distribution of subcutaneous fat in sportsmen: relationship to anaerobic power output (in preparation)

Watson, A. W. S. and D. J. O'Donovan (1976a) The reliability of measurements of physical working capacity, *Irish J. Med. Sci.* **145**: 308

Watson, A. W. S. and D. J. O'Donovan (1976b) The physical working capacity of male adolescents in Ireland, *Irish J. Med. Sci.* **145**: 383–91

Watson, A. W. S. and D. J. O'Donovan (1977a) Factors relating to the strength of male adolescents, *J. appl. Physiol.* **43**: 834–8

Watson, A. W. S. and D. J. O'Donovan (1977b) The effects of five weeks of controlled interval training on youths of diverse pre-training condition, *J. Sports Med.* **17**: 139–46

Watt, T., T. T. Romet, I. McEarlane, D. McGuey, C. Allen and R. C. Goode (1974) Vitamin E and oxygen consumption, *Lancet* **II**: 354–5

Weber, G., W. Kartodihardjo, and V. Klissouras (1976) Growth and physical training with special reference to heredity, *J. appl. Physiol.* **40**: 211–15

Wellock, L. M. (1958) Development of bilateral muscular strength through ipsilateral exercises, *Phys. Ther. Rev.* **35**: 671–5

Wilkerson, J. E. and E. Evonuk (1971) Changes in cardiac and skeletal muscle myosin ATP-ase activities after exercise, *J. appl. Physiol.* **30**: 328–30

Wilkie, D. R. (1959) Man as a source of mechanical power, *Ergonomics* **3**: 1–8

Wilkie, D. R. (1968) *Muscle*, London: Arnold

Williams, L. R. T. and V. Hearfield (1973) Heritability of a gross motor balance task, *Res. Quart.* **44**: 109–12

Williams, M. H. and A. J. Ward (1977) Hemotological changes elicited by prolonged intermittent aerobic exercise, *Res. Quart.* **48**: 606–16

Williams, R. (1976) *Skilful Rugby*, London: Souvenir Press

Wilmore, J., J. Davis, R. O'Brian, P. Vodak, G. Walder and E. Amsterdam (1975) A comparative investigation of bicycling, tennis and jogging as modes for altering cardiovascular endurance capacity, *Med. Sci. Sports* **7**: 83

Wilmore J. H., R. B. Parr, R. G. Girandola, P. Ward, P. Vodak, T. J. Barstow, T. V. Pipes, G. T. Romero and P. Leslie (1978) Physiological alterations to circuit weight training, *Med. Sci. Sports* **10**: 79–84

Withers, R. (1970) Effect of varied weight-training loads on the strength of university freshmen, *Res. Quart.* **41**: 110–14

Wolfe, L. A., D. A. Cunningham, P. Rechnitzer and P. M. Nichol (1979)

Effects of endurance training on left ventricular dimensions in healthy men, *J. appl. Physiol.* **47**: 207–12

Womersly, J. and J. V. G. A. Durnin (1973) An experimental study on variability of measurements of skinfold thickness on young adults, *Human Biology* **45**: 281–92

Wright, V. and R. J. Johns (1960) Physical factors concerned with the stiffness of normal and diseased joints, *John Hopkins Hospital Bull.* **106**: 215–31

Wyndham, C. H. (1967) Effect of acclimatisation on the sweat-rate/temperature relationship, *J. appl. Physiol.* **22**: 27–30

Wyndham, C. H. (1973) The physiology of exercise under heat stress, *Ann. Rev. Physiol.* **35**: 193–220

Young, D. R., R. Pelligra, J. Shapira, R. Adaehi and K. Skrettingland (1967) Glucose oxidation and replacement during prolonged exercise in man, *J. appl. Physiol.* **23**: 734–41

Zorbas, W. and P. Karpovich (1951) The effect of weightlifting upon the speed of muscular contractions, *Res. Quart.* **22**: 145–8

Zuntz, N., A. Loewy, F. Müller and W. Caspari (1906) *Hohenklima und Berg-wanderungen in ihrer Wirkung auf den Menschen*, Berlin: Deutsches Verlog-shaus Bong & Co.

INDEX